Controlled Release Pesticides

Controlled Release Pesticides

Herbert B. Scher, Editor
Stauffer Chemical Co.

A symposium sponsored by the Division of Pesticide Chemistry at the 173rd Meeting of the American Chemical Society, New Orleans, La., March 21–22, 1977.

ACS SYMPOSIUM SERIES **53**

AMERICAN CHEMICAL SOCIETY
WASHINGTON, D. C. 1977

Library of Congress CIP Data

Controlled release pesticides.

(ACS symopsium series; 53 ISSN 0097-6156)
Includes bibliographical references and index.

1. Pesticides, controlled release—Congresses.
I. Scher, Herbert B., 1937– II. American Chemical Society. Division of Pesticide Chemistry. III. Title. IV. Series: American Chemical Society. ACS symposium series; 53.

SB951.C648 1977 668'.65 77-22339
ISBN 0-8412-0382-2

PRINTED IN THE UNITED STATES OF AMERICA

ACS Symposium Series

Robert F. Gould, *Editor*

FOREWORD

The ACS Symposium Series was founded in 1974 to provide a medium for publishing symposia quickly in book form. The format of the Series parallels that of the continuing Advances in Chemistry Series except that in order to save time the papers are not typeset but are reproduced as they are submitted by the authors in camera-ready form. As a further means of saving time, the papers are not edited or reviewed except by the symposium chairman, who becomes editor of the book. Papers published in the ACS Symposium Series are original contributions not published elsewhere in whole or major part and include reports of research as well as reviews since symposia may embrace both types of presentation.

CONTENTS

PREFACE

Controlled release technology was pioneered by the drug industry approximately 25 years ago. The initial goal was to produce controlled release oral drug forms that could maintain an effective level of drug in the body, thereby eliminating the side effects caused by administrating high doses of conventional drugs. More recently, the drug industry has become even more sophisticated and has introduced controlled release drug forms capable of being implanted at the site of action, which further reduces drug levels and side effects.

Applying the same controlled release principles, pesticide scientists are now developing controlled release pesticide formulations capable of maintaining an effective level of pesticide in the soil or on foliage, thereby reducing pesticide application rates and minimizing pesticide levels in the environment. In addition, controlled release pesticide formulations can reduce pesticide toxicity and extend pesticide residual activity.

This volume is a compilation of information dealing with the structural and chemical factors governing the controlled release of pesticides from polymer systems. The first five papers deal with controlled release concepts, controlled release theory, and the environmental and toxicological aspects of controlled release pesticides. The next seven papers describe polymer systems that control the release of pesticides—i.e., elastomers, biodegradable matrices, polymers containing pendant pesticides, and microcapsules. The final four papers include research on microencapsulated insecticides for field use, laminated insecticide tapes for home use, a variety of systems for controlling the release of gypsy moth pheromone, and a microcapsule system for controlling the release of an insect growth regulator.

I would like to thank all the authors and J. J. Menn, J. P. Minyard, Jr., and G. G. Still of the Pesticide Division for their full cooperation during all phases of this symposium.

Richmond, Calif.
March 1977

HERBERT B. SCHER

1

Principles of Controlled Release Pesticides

D. H. LEWIS and D. R. COWSAR

Southern Research Institute, Birmingham, Ala. 35205

The rapidly growing demand for food and energy presents the scientific community with a major challenge. The need for more efficient operations in both industrial and agricultural production is paramount. Methods and processes that afford higher yields and better quality, require less time and money, and do not pose a threat to the environment are being sought at an unparalleled pace which undoubtedly will intensify further in the last quarter of this century. The control of pests, a battle fought for generations, is unquestionably a crucial task if our goals for the future concerning food and energy are to be achieved. Recent estimates suggest that losses due to inefficient pest-control techniques amount to between $10 and 30 billion each year (1). Losses of cotton alone to insects exceed $500 million per annum. (2) In India, rodents are reported (3) to destroy a fourth of the harvested grain crop annually. The astounding losses due to pests are not limited to food supplies alone. The fouling of ship hulls costs the U.S. Navy an additional $150 million/year in fuel (4), $15 million/year in labor and materials for repainting ships with antifoulants, and approximately $200 million each year for replacement of biologically deteriorated marine pilings (5). The importance of pesticides is evidenced by the estimated sale of $2.5 billion of pesticides each year in the U.S. alone (6). Although the reality of increasing danger to man from persistent pesticides is recognized, the frightening fact remains that if terrestrial herbicides alone were banned, starvation would become more prevalent in the world population in short order.

Historically, scientists have dealt with the problem of pest control by designing new, more potent agents. However, use of these agents to produce the desired biological response is often inefficient, primarily because of inabilities to deliver the agents to their targets at the precise time and in the optimum quantities required. Enormous amounts of funds are required for the development of a new biocide. Recent estimates place the development costs for a new pesticide at about $8 million (6). Recognizing the cost and limitations in the design of new pesticides, scientists began to turn in the 1960s to an alternative approach, that of improving the delivery of the agents, both newer agents and old.

In today's terminology, a controlled-release formulation or delivery system is defined as a combination of biologically active agent and excipient, usually a polymer, arranged to allow delivery of the agent to the target at controlled rates over a specified period. The rapid emergence of controlled release as an established scientific field is evidenced by the growing number of related publications appearing in the literature and the increasing number of symposia on the subject each year. As recent as 1973, for example, only one symposium was devoted to controlled release, while during 1976 several major meetings addressed the subject in depth. Few areas of research have activated the interest and attention of such a multidisciplinary group of professionals. Attendees at workshops, conferences, and symposia on controlled release typically include biologists, chemists, engineers, pharmacologists, agronomists, entomologists, veterinarians, dentists, and physicians. It is now a well recognized fact that the technology or controlled release can contribute positively to man's fight against disease and hunger.

Controlled release as applied to agricultural chemicals is fast becoming the subject of intensive research. Although slow-release fertilizers were known at least 30 years ago, most of the significant advances have come in the last 10 years. Obviously, in a field expanding so rapidly, a complete review of the literature cannot be given here. However, a number of excellent publications are available which offer more detailed treatments on fundamentals of controlled release and discussions of controlled-release pesticide formulations (7-12). Cardarelli (1), a pioneer in the field, has authored an excellent comprehensive review of controlled-release pesticide formulations. This chapter is intended to introduce the newcomer to the field, and for the experienced researcher, to make the papers that follow more cohesive. First, a brief discussion of the shortcomings of conventional methods of delivery will be given, then an overview of controlled-release formulations, and finally a few of the current applications of controlled release.

Advantages of Controlled Release

The principal advantage of controlled-release formulations is that they allow much less pesticide to be used for the same period of activity. Moreover, when the normal half-life of a potent pesticide is short, the release formulations are especially advantageous in comparison to conventional methods of application. To fully understand this benefit, one must first understand the magnitude of the environmental forces that act to remove excesses of pesticides from their sites of application.

When applied by conventional methods, pesticides are invariably subject to leaching, evaporation, and degradation (photolytic, hydrolytic, and microbial), all of which remove the active materials from their target before they can perform their function. In most cases, the rate of removal follows first-order kinetics, *i.e.*, the rate of removal at any time is directly proportional to the amount (or concentration of the pesticide present in the environment at that time. A mathematical expression of the first-order rate law is given by Equation 1,

$$\frac{dM}{dt} = -k_r M_t \qquad (1)$$

where dM/dt is the rate of removal, k_r is the rate constant, and M_t is the amount of pesticide present at any time t. The integrated solution to Equation 1 is

$$\ln\left(\frac{M_t}{M_\infty}\right) = -k_r t \qquad (2)$$

where M_∞ is the amount present at $t = 0$; M_∞ is thus the amount applied. The rate of removal of a pesticide from the environment is often expressed as the agent's half-life, $t_{1/2}$. The half-life is related to the first-order rate constant for removal, k_r, as follows:

$$\ln 2 = -k_r t_{1/2} \qquad (3)$$

or,

$$k_r = \ln 2/t_{1/2} = 0.693/t_{1/2} \qquad (4)$$

If M_e is the minimum effective level of pesticide and M_∞ is the amount of agent applied initially, then the time, t_e, during which an effective level of pesticide is present after a single application is given by Equation 5.

$$\ln\left(\frac{M_\infty}{M_e}\right) = k_r t_e \qquad (5)$$

From Eq. 5, it follows that to increase the effective duration of action, t_e, of a conventionally applied pesticide, exponentially greater quantities of the pesticide must be applied. On the other hand, if the pesticide could be maintained at the minimum effective level, M_e, by a continuous supply to restore the fraction dissipated, then the optimum performance of a pesticide would be realized when the instantaneous rate of removal equals the instantaneous rate of delivery,

$$\frac{dM}{dt} = -k_r M_e + k_d M_e = 0 \qquad (6)$$

In Equation 6, k_d is the rate constant for pesticide delivery. When a pesticide is formulated for sustained delivery, the duration of action, t_e, of the formulation is given by Equation 7.

$$\frac{M_\infty - M_e}{M_e} = k_d t_e \qquad (7)$$

Figure 1 shows the relationships between the level of application and the duration of action for conventional first-order formulations (Equation 5 is plotted as Curve A) and for controlled-release formulations (Equation 7 is plotted as Curve B). In preparing Figure 1, we assumed that the half-life of the pesticide was 15 days and that the minimum effective level was 1 g/acre. To achieve protection for 50 days with a conventional formulation (Curve A), the level of application would have to increase tenfold, but only a third of the pesticide would be used to control the target organism. For double and triple this duration of action, the levels of pesticide applied must be multiplied by a hundred and a thousand, respectively. For an optimized controlled-release formulation (Curve B), the amounts needed for 50, 100, and 150 days of pest control are, respectively, 3.3, 5.6, and 7.9 g of the active material. The area between Curves A and B on the logarithmic scale represents the fraction of conventional pesticide applied which serves no useful purpose; hence, it is wasted. Moreover, the magnitude of the amount wasted is increased substantially if the half-life of the conventional biocide is shorter than our arbitrary 15 days.

Obviously, the pesticides already in use can be improved to minimize the waste of these costly and toxic chemicals, which may later cause an ecologic catastrophy, and to extend the duration of action of safer, less-persistent analogs. The key is the design and development of sustained-delivery devices and formulations. The extent to which optimum results are achievable depends primarily on the degree to which the factors affecting the rate and duration of release of pesticides from sustained-delivery systems can be controlled precisely.

Mechanisms of Controlled Release

Controlled release is not synonymous with sustained release, a much older and well recognized concept from which the new science is emerging, although the two are similar in principle and sometimes overlap. Sustained-release formulations are so-called because they contain several times the normal single application, and they provide for replacement of the agent at some rate which gives a measurable increase in the duration of activity. The rate may decrease due to gradual loss of agent, or increase through a maximum due to breakdown of a protective barrier. A controlled-release formulation, in contrast, may exhibit a fast or a slow release, or a constant or a changing release, depending on the design. The principal difference lies not entirely in the profiles of release but in the mechanism of release. The distinction is drawn mainly by the degree of control of both the optimum level and the optimum time of availability of the biologically active agent.

The concept and practice of controlled release encompasses many mechanisms. Although the earliest formulations were based on the desorption of pesticides from strong sorbents like silica gel, mica, and activated charcoal (13), most of the current systems are based on more controllable mechanisms such as diffusion through rate-controlling media, erosion of biodegradable barrier materials, and retrograde chemical reactions. Designers of controlled-release formulations or devices usually strive for zero-order (constant) rates of release, but systems with time-dependent release kinetics are proving to be useful for pesticides, especially when the rate and duration of release are predictable and well controlled. In practice, the rate of pesticide release may be controlled by several sequential or simultaneous mechanisms which do not lend themselves to simple analysis, but it is usually possible to determine

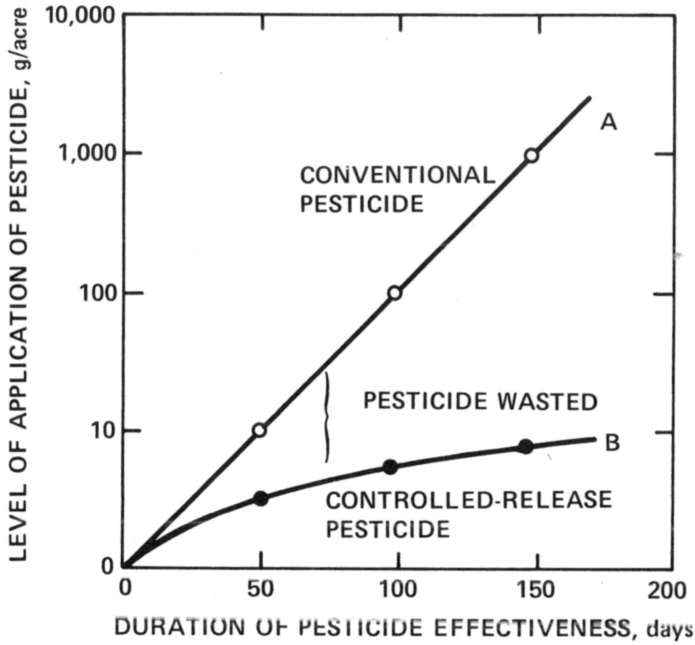

Figure 1. Relationships between the level of application and the duration of action for conventional and controlled release formulations

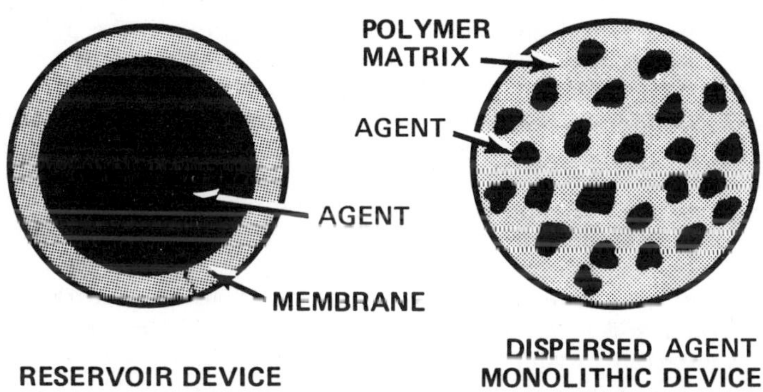

Figure 2. Reservoir and monolithic diffusion controlled devices

experimentally an overall "apparent" order of release for these complex systems.

Many design concepts have been studied in development of controlled-release formulations for pesticides. Three of the most promising ones are the following: (1) capsules of polymeric material filled with a solid or liquid pesticide or with a suspension or solution of the agent in a fluid, in which the release of pesticide is controlled by Fickian diffusion through the capsule walls or through micropores in the capsule walls; (2) a heterogeneous dispersion of particles or droplets of pesticide in a solid polymeric matrix, which can be either biodegradable or nonbiodegradable and which controls the release of agent by diffusion through the matrix, by erosion of the matrix, or by a combination of both diffusion and erosion; and (3) chemical bonding of a pesticide to a natural or synthetic polymeric material, as by pendant anhydride or ester linkages, or formation of macromolecules of pesticides via ionic or covalent linkages, which control the release of the agent by hydrolysis, thermodynamic dissocation, microbial degradation, or some other retrograde chemical reaction of the linkages.

Release by membrane-moderated diffusion. Diffusion-controlled membrane devices can be divided into two main categories: reservoir systems in which the pesticide is totally encapsulated within a rate-controlling membrane, and monolithics systems in which the pesticide is dispersed or dissolved in a rate-controlling matrix. These systems are depicted in Figure 2. It has been demonstrated that the diffusion rates from controlled-release systems follow Fick's law of diffusion, which states that the rate of diffusion depends on five factors. Two of the factors involve the geometry or dimensions of the device, and three involve pesticide-polymer interactions.

$$\frac{dM}{dt} = \frac{A}{h} D(C_s - KC_e) \tag{8}$$

In Equation 8, the dimensional factors are A, the surface area of the membrane; and h, the thickness through which diffusion occurs. The diffusional factors are D, the diffusion coefficient of the pesticide in the polymer; C_s, the saturation solubility of the pesticide in the polymer; and K, the partition coefficient of the pesticide between the polymer and the medium which surrounds the device. C_e in Equation 8 is the concentration of released pesticide in the environment. The solubility and the partition coefficient are susceptible to analysis and prediction in terms of appropriate thermodynamic solution theories. The mobility of the penetrant pesticide molecules, as measured by the diffusion coefficient, is a kinetic parameter governed by the size, shape, and polarity of the penetrant and by the morphology of the diffusion medium.

When applied to reservoir systems, Fick's law predicts that if a pesticide is enclosed within an inert membrane, and if the concentration is maintained constant within the enclosure, then a steady state will be established during which the release rate will be zero order, i.e, constant. The various forms of Fick's law which apply to reservoir systems of familiar geometries are given in Figure 3 for the slab or laminate device and for the sphere or microcapsule.

Membrane-moderated monolithic systems in which the pesticide is dispersed or dissolved in a rate-controlling polymer matrix are simple to prepare, but they do not have the zero-order release kinetics of the reservoir systems. The pesticide is released from the surface layers of a monolithic device first, and the distance the pesticide must diffuse to reach the surface increases with time. Thus, these systems have slowly declining rates of release. The kinetics of release can follow two patterns depending on whether the pesticide is present as a solution or as a dispersion.

For delivery of pesticide which has been dissolved in a spherical polymer bead of radius r_o, the expressions of Fick's law which describe the rate of release are given by Equations 9 and 10.

$$\frac{dM_t/M_\infty}{dt} = 6\left(\frac{Dt}{r_o^{\,2}\pi}\right)^{1/2} - \frac{3Dt}{r_o^{\,2}} \tag{9}$$

$$\frac{dMt/M_\infty}{dt} = 1 - \frac{6}{\pi^2}\exp\left(\frac{-\pi^2 Dt}{r_o^{\,2}}\right) \tag{10}$$

Equation 9 is called the "early-time approximation" and is valid for $M_t/M_\infty < 0.5$, and Equation 10 is called the "late-time approximation" and is valid for $M_t/M_\infty > 0.5$. From these equations it is apparent that about the first 50% of the pesticide is released at a rate which decreases as the square root of time, and the rate of release of remaining pesticide follows exponential of first-order kinetics. Figure 4 depicts these equations graphically. Equations for the slab and cylindrical geometries have also been derived (14).

If the pesticide is dispersed in the spherical polymer matrix rather than dissolved, the release kinetics are altered, and the rate of release is described by Equation 11.

$$\frac{dM_t/M_\infty}{dt} = \frac{3C_sD}{r_o^{\,2}C_o}\left[\frac{(1-M_t/M_\infty)^{1/3}}{1-(1-M_t/M_\infty)^{1/3}}\right] \tag{11}$$

This equation is valid as long as the total amount of pesticide in the matrix C_o is much larger than the saturation solubility of pesticide in the matrix, C_s. Figure 5 shows the release profiles of monolithic devices with different initial loadings. It is not possible in this case to express the release rate as a single function of time. If, however, Equation 11 is integrated, an expression of the time, t_∞, required for the spherical beads to become totally exhausted of dispersed pesticide can be derived as shown in Equation 12.

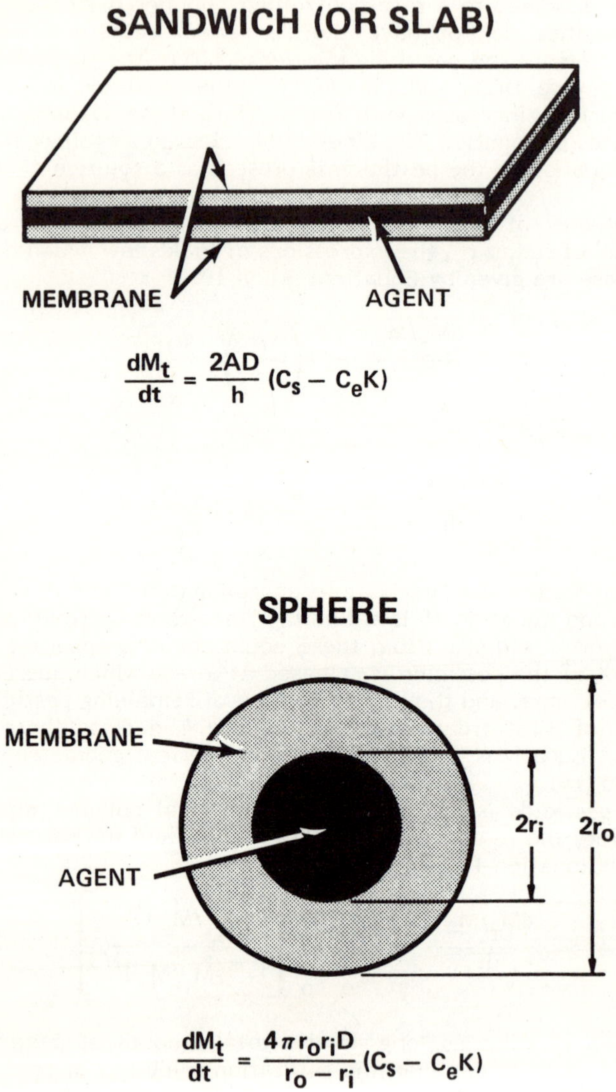

Figure 3. Expressions of Fick's law for reservoir devices

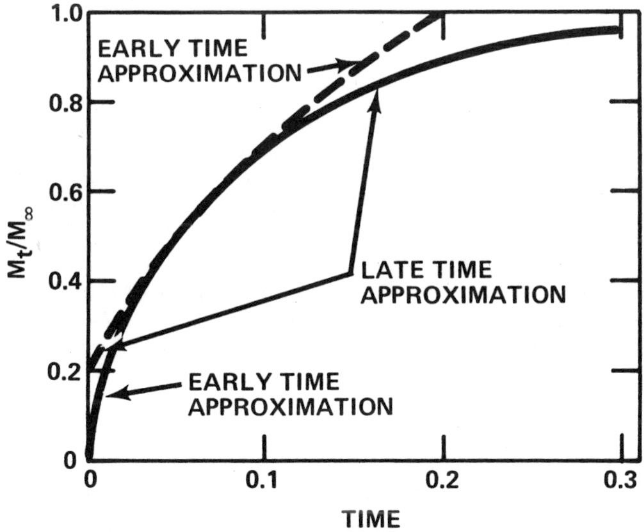

Figure 4. Fraction of agent desorbed from a monolithic device as a function of time

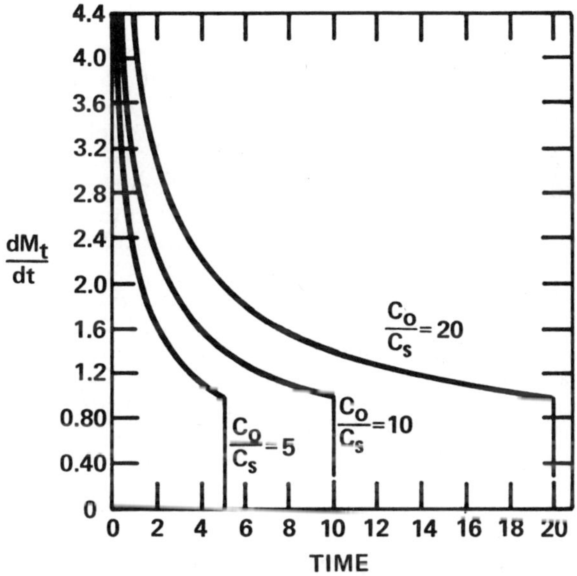

Figure 5. Release profiles of monolithic devices with different initial loadings of dispersed agent

$$t_\infty = \frac{r_o^2 C_o}{6 DC_s} \qquad (12)$$

Release by erosion. When the polymer containing dispersed or dissolved pesticide is water soluble, hydrolytically unstable, or otherwise biodegradable, the active material can be released by diffusion of the pesticide from the polymer, by erosion of the polymer, or by a combination of both diffusion and erosion. Release by erosion is a surface-area-dependent phenomenon, and if the surface area of a device stays constant while it is eroding, the release of pesticide will be zero order. The general expression which the describes the rate of release by a purely erosion mechanism is given in Equation 13,

$$\frac{dM_t}{dt} = k_E C_o A \qquad (13)$$

where k_E is the erosion rate constant, A is the surface area exposed to the environment, and C_o is the loading of pesticide in the erodible matrix.

For the flat film or slab geometry, the surface area does not change as erosion occurs, and consequently, the release of agent is constant until the film ultimately disappears. For an erodible sphere or radius r_o, the rate of release of pesticide is given by Equation 14.

$$\frac{dM_t}{dt} = 4\pi\, C_o k_E (r_o - k_E t)^2 \qquad (14)$$

It is apparent from this equation that pesticide release decreases slowly with time, and that zero-order kinetics are not possible with spherical systems of this type.

If the pesticide is contained as a single reservoir within a spherical bioerodible membrane, as in some microcapsules, the mechanism of release can be the erosion and rupture of the barrier membrane. Various delivery patterns, including essentially constant release, can be achieved by blending microcapsules of appropriate wall thicknesses.

Release by retrograde chemical reactions. As opposed to physical combinations of pesticides dissolved or entrapped in polymers, chemical combinations have the pesticide firmly attached to the polymeric substrate by a definite identifiable chemical bond. The active material is released when environmental reactants such as water, air, sunlight, or microorganisms act to cleave the specific chemical linkages which attach the pesticide to the substrate. The general mechanism for retrograde chemical systems is shown in Equation 15.

$$\text{Polymer} + \text{Pesticide} \underset{\text{environment}}{\overset{\text{synthesis}}{\rightleftharpoons}} \text{Polymeric Pesticide} \qquad (15)$$

Obviously, only those pesticides with at least one reactive functional moiety can be utilized in delivery systems of this type. The most common linkages are esters, anhydrides, and acetals.

The rate of release of pesticides via retrograde reactions depends on the properties of the macromolecule and its surrounding medium. When water present in the environment is used to activate the release of pesticide, the rate of hydrolysis depends on the strength and chemical nature of the polymer pesticide bond. For example, an anhydride linkage is more susceptible than an ester or amide linkage to hydrolysis. The rate of hydrolysis of a linkage is also dependent on the groups surrounding it. Hydrophobic groups thus offer protection against rapid hydrolysis. An uncrosslinked polymer is much more susceptible to hydrolysis than a highly crosslinked one, and a stereoregular or crystalline polymer is less susceptible to hydrolytic attack than an amorphous or atactic polymer.

The kinetic expressions which describe the rate of release of pesticides from retrograde chemical systems vary depending on whether the hydrolysis reaction, for example, occurs on the surface of an insoluble particle or in solution. For a heterogeneous reaction on the surface of insoluble spherical particles, the rate of release of pesticide is given by Equation 16,

$$\frac{dM_t}{dt} = nk_h 4\pi r_o^2 C_o \qquad (16)$$

where h is the number of particles of average radius r_o, k_n is the reaction rate constant for hydrolysis, and C_o is the concentration of pesticide-polymer linkages. For water-soluble delivery systems, the rate of release of pendant pesticide groups follows conventional first-order kinetics. Finally, retrograde chemical systems which are based on depolymerization reactions may indeed be zero order if the mechanism of release comprises unzipping of polymer chains.

Applications

Membrane-moderated diffusion systems for home use were some of the first contolled-release pesticides to be marketed. The Hercon Lure 'N Kill™ Fly Tape and Roach-Tape® are laminated reservoir devices developed by the Health Chem Corporation (15). The Hercon strips comprise agent-containing reservoirs sandwiched between layers of plastic film. The outer plastic film serves as a membrane to control the release of pesticide from the reservoir. The Hercon fly strip is probably the first such product to combine an insecticide with an insect attractant. Resmethrin, the active ingredient in the Lure 'N Kill™ Fly Tape, kills by direct contact rather than by vapors. The product is reported to be effective for at least three months. The Shell No-Pest Strip® is another widely used controlled-release product. Since dichlorvos, the active insecticide, is codissolved with a plasticizer in the PVC matrix, the No-Pest Strip is a monolith device, and the release rate decreases with the square root of time.

NoFoul® Rubber developed and marketed by the B. F. Goodrich Company has proven successful as an antifouling coating (6 - 8). The product releases bis(tri-n-butyltin)oxide (TBTO) which is dissolved at a level of 2 to 5% in Neoprene rubber. After extensive evaluations, the NoFoul product has proven to be effective for periods of up to 92 months. Cardarelli and his coworkers (17, 18) have been responsible for many of the advances made in controlled-release antifoulant systems.

Beginning around 1968, a number of systems for delivering aquatic herbicides were investigated. Cardarelli (1) incorporated the butoxyethanol ester of 2,4-D(2,4-D BEE) in a variety of polymers including natural rubber. The primary mechanism of release of that herbicide from the natural rubber matrix was membrane-moderated diffusion of agent dissolved in the monolith since 2,4-D-BEE is 35 to 40% soluble in natural rubber. Carbon black was used to slow the release of agent. The particle size, structure, and amount of carbon black were shown to be critical. A variety of formulations, termed sinkers or floaters, were developed to allow agent to be released at the water surface or at predetermined depths. Field tests have shown the duration of action of the system to be about two years. Young and Nelson incorporated a number of 2,4-D derivatives including 2,4-D BEE in plasticized PVC (19). The mechanism of release from those formulations appeared to be codiffusion of plasticizers and agents. Harris (20) has prepared a series of diffusion-type delivery systems by dispersing the herbicide Fenac® (sodium salt of 2,3,6-trichlorophenylacetic acid) in porous polyethylene matrixes.

Microencapsulation techniques have been used to prepare spherical-shaped reservoir devices for controlled release of pesticides. The most often-used procedures include phase separation, coacervation, spray coating, solvent evaporation from emulsions, and interfacial polymerizations. The choice of method depends mainly upon the characteristics of the pesticide and release-controlling membrane. Common polymeric wall materials include polyamides, polyesters, polyureas, cellulose, and gelatin.

The most notable of the currently marketed microcapsule products is probably the Penncap-M formulation developed by the Pennwalt Corporation (21, 22). The short-acting pesticide, methyl parathion, is encapsulated in a polyamide (nylon) wall material. The microcapsules are about 30 microns in diameter, and they contain about 80% of the active agent by weight. This product, which has received registration with the Environmental Protection Agency, exhibits decreased toxicity and longer activity when compared with the conventional application of the insecticide.

The 3M Company markets a line of fertilizers microencapsulated in polymeric membranes. These are primarily speciality products for home use such as the Precise Timed-Release Plant Food, the Precise Timed-Release African Violet Food, among others. Release of the agent occurs by controlled diffusion through the capsule walls and the duration of action is 3 to 6 months.

In addition to these delivery systems which operate by diffusion or leaching mechanisms, other formulations which rely on erosion or a combination of erosion and diffusion have been reported.

Sinclair (23) demonstrated that solid agents could be mixed with a polymeric material and extruded or pressed into pellets which would then deliver the agent at a slow rate. The sodium salt of 2,4-D was mixed with pulverized poly(lactic acid) (PLA), and the resulting mixture was pressed into pellets. The slow-release characteristics of the pellets, determined in vitro in moist sandy soil, showed that 70% of the agent was released in about 20 days, with 25% being dumped on the first day. Erosion of the PLA and leaching of the solubilized agent governed the release of the herbicide.

A series of solid and liquid pesticides was recently microencapsulated in starch xanthate by Shasha and coworkers (24). The mechanism of release from the starch capsules was a combination of diffusion and erosion. Incorporation of a small amount of latex rubber with the starch xanthate slowed the release of pesticide from the system, but they did not determine whether the latex inhibited diffusion or erosion.

One of the first microencapsulated pesticides to be introduced was Tossits®, a DDT product marketed by the Wyco International Company. The DDT/oil mixture in the core of the gelatin-walled capsules was dumped when the walls of the microcapsules ruptured. The Wurster coating process (25) has been used to prepare a number of erosion-controlled formulations. Warfin, coated in that manner, is more effective as a rodenticide since the coating serves to mask the taste of the bait until it is injested. The time of release is controlled since the rodenticide is released in the rat's stomach.

An increasingly attractive approach to designing new controlled-release systems is that of attaching the agent by covalent or ionic bonds to a polymer chain as pendent groups. In most of the formulations of this type reported thus far, the principle mechanism of release is hydrolysis of a covalent linkage between the pendent pesticide group and the backbone of the polymer. Allan (26, 27) and coworkers were among the first to report the synthesis and evaluation of various polymers containing pendent herbicide moities. Recently, Harris et al prepared a series of homopolymers and copolymers with pendant herbicide substituents (28, 29). The 2-acryloyloxyethyl esters of 2,4-D and Silvex were copolymerized with comonomers such as trimethylamine methacrylimide and acrylic acid. Their studies showed that the rate of hydrolysis of connecting ester linkages can be greatly enhanced by the incorporation of aminimide or carboxylic groups along the polymer chain.

In a novel approach, Neogi and Allan (30, 31) combined monomeric herbicides with bark from the Douglas Fir tree. One herbicide, 2,4-dichlorophenoxy-γ-butyric acid, was esterified with the bark to produce about 37% of releasable agent. The herbicide was applied at several levels in a 25-ft diameter circle around Douglas Fir seedlings. Data obtained after 4 years show that trees treated with the controlled-release formulation are growing 16% faster per year than the untreated trees. In addition to the developments of herbicides reported by Allan and Harris, advances have been made with various antifouling agents in a similar approach. U.S. Navy researchers (4, 32) have successfully incorporated organotin units as pendent groups along the backbone of addition polymers. The most promising formulations appear to be those with ester linkages between the pesticide and the polymer backbone. As with the herbicides, the primary mode of release is hydrolysis of the ester group. Field trials of formulations developed by the Navy indicate up to 4 years of 100% resistance to all forms of fouling (4).

The ideal controlled-release pesticide system would probably be one in which the active agent was generated as needed from a macromolecular structure of the agent itself. In other words, the monomeric pesticide would be homopolymerized to a high-molecular-weight substance which upon hydrolysis, thermodynamic dissociation, or microbial degradation would yield active agent. Or perhaps a comonomer could be used which would not be detrimental if released to the environment. Very little research and development has been reported in this area. Neogi in 1970 (33) prepared a number of condensation polymers which contained pesticides in the polymer chain. We are aware of no other successful attempts to formulate a pesticide-releasing system of this type.

Other controlled-release systems are based on concepts somewhat different from those previously discussed. Hollow fibers have been used to deliver biologically active agents for extended periods. The FRL Corporation developed the Conrel® Hollow-Fiber Controlled-Release Strips (34, 35). The active agent is contained within the lumen of a small-diameter hollow fiber usually made of polyester. The release of agent is a three-step mechanism: evaporation at the liquid-vapor interface, diffusion to the open end of the fiber, and convection away from the open end. The Conrel® system has been tested for delivery of behavioral chemicals such as endo- and exo-brevicomin for control of the Southern Pine Bettle. The agents were released at nearly constant rates of 3.0 mg/day over a 30-day period. The hollow-fiber dispenser has proven useful in the mass trapping of a number of other insects with phenomones.

Steward and coworkers (36) recently reported field trials with a water-in-oil emulsion which delivers the aquatic herbicide, Diquat, over prolonged periods. The most promising systems were formulated with diesel oils as the organic phase; they contained a number of emulsifiers and stabilizers. The addition of triethanolamine/copper complexes increased the efficacy of the Diquat formulations.

One should recognize that many pesticides are not amenable to administration by controlled-release formulations or devices, and others can be delivered equally effectively by simple alternative means. It must also be emphasized that each agent usually requires a delivery system designed specifically for the agent and the intended application. Unfortunately, considerable amounts of time and funds have often been expended in unsuccessful attempts to formulate acceptable delivery systems from so-called general or universal procedures. If the numerous potential advantages of controlled release are to be fully realized, the researcher must select and formulate the best system possible for the particular end use.

Literature Cited

1. Cardarelli, N. F., "Controlled Release Pesticides Formulations", CRC Press, Inc., Cleveland, Ohio, 1976.

2. Marx, J. L., Science, (1977), 195, 860.
3. Anon., Wildlife Research Laboratory Report, U.S. Dept. of the Interior, Denver, 1969.
4. Castelli, V. J. and Yeager, W. L., in "Controlled Release Polymeric Formulations", D. R. Paul and F. W. Harris, eds., pp. 239-247, ACS Symposium Series 33, American Chemical Society, Washington, D.C., 1976.
5. Fischer, E. C., in "Proceedings 1976 International Controlled Release Pesticide Symposium", N. F. Cardarelli, ed., University of Akron, Akron, Ohio, 1976.
6. Ovellete, R. P. and King, J., Chemical Week, June 23, 1976, p. 27.
7. Tanquary, A. C. and Lacey, R. E., eds., "Controlled Release of Biologically Active Agents", Plenum Press, New York, 1974.
8. Cardarelli, N. F., ed., "Proceedings Controlled Release Pesticide Symposium", University of Akron, Akron, Ohio, 1974.
9. Harris, F. W., ed., "Proceedings Controlled Release Pesticide Symposium", Wright State University, Dayton, Ohio, 1975.
10. Cardarelli, N. F., ed., "Proceedings 1976 Controlled Release Pesticide Symposium", University of Akron, Akron, Ohio, 1976.
11. Paul, D. R. and Harris, F. W., eds., "Controlled Release Polymeric Formulations", ACS Symposium Series 33, American Chemical Society, Washington, D.C., 1976.
12. Baker, R. W. and Lonsdale, H. K., Chemtech, (1975), 5, 668.
13. Caprio, A. F. and Horback, W., U.S. Patent 2,460,376, February 1, 1949.
14. Baker, R. W. and Lonsdale, H. K., in "Controlled Release of Biologically Active Agents", A. C. Tanquary and R. E. Lacey, eds., pp. 15-61, Plenum Press, New York, 1974.
15. Quisumbing, A. R., Kydonieus, A. F., Calsett, D. R., and Haus, J. B., in "Proceedings 1976 Controlled Release Pesticide Symposium", N. F. Cardarelli, ed., University of Akron, Akron, Ohio, 1976.
16. Phillip, A.T., Prog. Org. Coat., (1973), 2, 159.
17. Cardarelli, N. F. and Neff, H . F., French Patent 1, 506,704 (1966).
18. Cardarelli, N. F. and Neff, H. F., U.S. Patent 3,639,583, (1972).
19. Young, W. W. and Nelson, L. L., "Evaluation of controlled release herbicide formulations for aquatic weeds", Special Study No. 31-004-69/70. Dept. of the Army, U.S. Army Environmental Hygiene Agency, Edgewood Arsenal, Md., 1969.
20. Harris, F. W., Norris, S. V., and Post, L. K., Weed Sci., (1973), 21, 318.
21. Koeslter, R. C. and Ivy, E. E. in "Proceedings Controlled Release Pesticide Symposium", N. F. Cardarelli, ed., University of Akron, Akron, Ohio, 1974.
22. Koeslter, R. C., in "Proceedings 1976 Controlled Release Pesticide Symposium", N. F. Cardarelli, ed., University of Akron, Akron, Ohio, 1976.
23. Sinclair, R. G., Environmental Science and Technology, (1973), 7, 955.
24. Shasha, B. S., Doane, W. M., and Russell, C. R., J. Poly. Sci., Polymer Letters Edition, (1976), 14, 417.

25. Anon., "The Wurster Air Suspension Process for Encapsulation", Wisconsin Alumni Research Foundation, Coating Laboratory Report, Middleton, Wisconsin, 1974.
26. Allan, G. G., Chopra, C. S., Neogi, A. N., and Wilkins, R. M., Tappi, (1971), 54, 1293.
27. Allan, G. G., Chopra, C. S., Friedloff, J. F., Gara, R. I., Maggi, M. W., Neogi, A. N., Roberts, S. C., and Wilkins, R. W., Chem. Tech., (1973), March, 171.
28. Harris, F. W. and Post, L. K., J. Poly. Sci., Polymer Letters Edition, (1975), 13, 225.
29. Harris, F. W., Aulabaugh, A. E., Case, R. D., Dykes, M. K., and Field, W. A., in "Controlled Release Polymeric Formulations", D. R. Paul and F. W. Harris, eds., ACS Symposium Series Number 33, pp. 222-230, American Chemical Society, Washington, D.C.
30. Neogi, A. N. and Allan, C. G., in "Controlled Release of Biologically Active Agents", A. C. Tanquary and R. E. Lacey, eds., pp. 195-224, Plenum Press, New York, 1974.
31. Allan, G. G., Cousin, M. J., McConnell, W. J., Powell, J. C., and Yahiaoui, A., in "Proceedings 1976 Controlled Release Pesticide Symposium", N. F. Cardarelli, ed., University of Akron, Akron, Ohio, 1976.
32. Dyckman, E. J., Montemarano, J. A., and Fischer, E. C., Nav. Eng. J., (1973), 85, 33.
33. Neogi, A. N., "Polymer Selection for Controlled Release Pesticides", Ph.D. Thesis, University of Washington, 1970.
34. Ashare, E., Brooks, T. W., and Swenson, D. W., in "Proceedings Con trolled Release Pesticide Symposium", F. W. Harris, ed., Wright State University.
35. Payne, T. L., Coster, J. E., Johnson, P. C., in "Proceedings 1976 Controlled Release Pesticide Symposium", N. F. Cardarelli, ed., University of Akron, Akron, Ohio, 1976.
36. Steward, K. K., Jones, A. O., and Hayl, C. J., in Proceedings 1976 Controlled Release Pesticide Symposium", N. F. Cardarelli, ed., University of Akron, Akron, Ohio, 1976.

2

Structural and Chemical Factors Controlling the Permeability of Organic Molecules through a Polymer Matrix

C. E. ROGERS

Department of Macromolecular Science, Case Western Reserve University, Cleveland, Ohio 44106

The use of polymeric materials in controlled release application systems almost always involves consideration of the solubility and diffusivity of the active agent in the polymer matrix. The configuration of the release system, be it reservoir-type or a simple dispersal of dissolved agent (we exclude any specific discussion of polymer degradation release systems), is of little significance in this context. In certain systems there may be a rate-controlling step related to interfacial processes which affect the attainment of equilibrium across a reservoir-membrane phase boundary apart from normal boundary layer phenomena. Except for such uncommon situations, the release rate characteristics of the system will reflect the diffusion rates, solution levels, and resultant gradients of dissolved and diffusing agent within the controlling polymer membrane.

The inherent nature of transport processes in polymeric media can be explained and predicted in terms of established models, theories, and phenomenological observations. There is an extensive literature which deals with the solution, diffusion, and permeation of low molecular weight gases, vapors, liquids, and ions in polymer films (1-6). Unfortunately, there are relatively few studies involving the transport characteristics of larger organic molecules in polymers. This, in large part, is due to the experimental difficulties involved in such investigations. Pertinent data relating to the solubility and migration of larger molecules in polymers can be gleaned from the literature dealing with controlled release systems (7-16), encapsulation (17-23), and plasticizer technology.

The nature of solution, diffusion, and permeation behavior in all membrane systems is common insofar as those processes and other properties of the materials are governed by the physiochemical composition and structure of the components under given environmental conditions. The phenomena of controlled release are similar (often identical) to those involved in plasticizer technology, coatings technology, environmental resistance of polymers, and related areas of polymer technology. The extensive investigations in those areas can serve as both theoretical and practical guides in the development of controlled release systems.

An important consideration leading to an elucidation of solution and diffusion behavior in many controlled release applications is that the polymeric matrix often is modified upon exposure to the application environment. Examples of common modifications are changes in polymer structure and morphology due to changes in temperature or pH and changes in polymer density and homogeniety of structural packing due to swelling caused by an imbided environmental species such as water. Other major complications affecting controlled release systems, such as boundary layer phenomena and/or membrane fouling, are well recognized. Consequently, it is a challenge to either alleviate the seriousness of these effects or, perhaps even better, to turn them to some advantage. In any case, an understanding of the nature of solution and diffusion processes and their dependence on penetrant, polymer, and environmental factors is a key element in the design of viable polymer membrane controlled release systems.

With these concepts in mind, we will discuss aspects of the general dependence of diffusion and solution processes on certain structural factors. We wish to emphasize a few underlying principles and phenomena common to many types of application and to suggest avenues to approach the solution of remaining problem areas. In particular, we want to call attention to aspects of the general concentration dependence of solution/diffusion processes which seem to be both neglected (or misunderstood) and promising for the development of effective controlled release systems.

Factors Affecting Membrane Permeability

The mechanism of transport of a penetrant agent within a polymeric material can be classified in terms of the presence or absence of a) a gross porous (or highly swollen) structure and b) fixed ionic charges. In the first case, the transport behavior is closely governed by the relative molecular dimensions of the penetrant as compared to the pore diameter and connectivity. This mechanism is dominant in dialysis and ultrafiltration membrane systems. The electrostatic interactions between the penetrant molecule and the polymer-fixed ionic groups, as modified by the action of other sorbed species, is a dominant factor in ion exchange and some biological membrane systems.

In the absence of the above overriding factors, the most common mechanism of transport is the solution-diffusion model. In this case, the overall transport process depends on a multitude of factors relating to such aspects as the size, shape, composition, and concentration of the penetrant and the polymer composition, structure, and morphology. Although the number of factors, and interactions between factors, may lead to complex relationships to describe the solution-diffusion behavior, it is this complexity which can allow us to design and develop unique and useful membrane systems.

Regardless of the state of aggregation of the mixture, the diffusion flow or flux, J, of a substance in a mixture with other substances can be defined as the amount passing during unit time through a surface of unit area normal to the direction of flow. In many cases of interest for release applications, it is necessary to realize that the total flux may be a combination of a pure diffusive flux and other fluxes due to mass flow, flow through defects, or flow due to externally imposed stress or other driving force. Suitable corrections to account for the frame of reference for such systems have been discussed (2,3,5). The concepts and procedures of irreversible thermodynamics are generally applicable. These corrections seldom have been made in practice so that the interpretation of most published data is subject to reappraisal in terms of interferences which are made on the basis of concepts and theories for diffusive mechanisms of transport.

The flux in the steady-state (or pseudo-steady-state over relatively short time periods) for corrected pure diffusive flux can be expressed as:

$$J = -DK(dc/dx) = -D^*(d\ln a/d\ln\bar{c})(d\bar{c}/dc)(dc/dx) \quad (1)$$

where $DK = \underline{P}$, the permeability constant. The diffusion coefficient D^* is a measure of the average mobility of penetrant molecules within the diffusion medium. The distribution factor (solubility coefficient)

$$K = (d\bar{c}/dc) \quad (2)$$

is a measure of the partitioning of penetrant between a polymer solution phase, $\bar{c}$, and an ambient penetrant phase, c. The latter phase may be the phase external to the membrane, the enclosed penetrant reservoir, or dispersed phase-separated penetrant "micro-reservoirs" within the polymeric matrix. The Nernst-type distribution function is a thermodynamic parameter characterizing the penetrant-polymer system which can be a function of pressure or concentration as well as temperature.

The apparent Fick's Law diffusion coefficient, D, is the product of the non-negative mobility factor and a thermodynamic factor related to the ideality of the penetrant-polymer mixture:

$$D = D^*(d\ln a/d\ln\bar{c}) \quad (3)$$

where a is the activity and $\bar{c}$ is the concentration of penetrant in solution in the polymer phase. When the mixture is a thermodynamically ideal solution, $d\ln a/d\ln\bar{c}$ is unity. However, most mixtures exhibit deviations from ideal behavior of a magnitude proportional to the concentration.

The thermodynamic term also can be expressed as

$$d\ln a/d\ln\bar{c} = 1 + (d\ln\gamma/d\ln\bar{c}) \qquad (4)$$

where γ is the activity coefficient. If, for any reason, the thermodynamic term becomes negative in sign, diffusion occurs against the concentration gradient. The presence of unstable phase regions within the diffusion medium, due, for example, to sudden local changes in applied stress or temperature, will lead to this "uphill" diffusion behavior which is phenomenologically similar to "activated" transport in biological systems.

The concentration dependence of D is seen to arise from two sources: the concentration dependence of the mobility, usually the dominant factor, and a concentration dependence attributed to the non-ideal nature of the system, per se. These factors can be interpreted and assessed in terms of theories or models concerned with polymer solution behavior, the mode of sorption, molecular friction factors, chain segmental mobility, free volume concepts, etc. Certain of these aspects will be described in a later section.

It is well to note that the definitions of K and D do not impose any restrictions as to the functional dependence of the parameters on experimental conditions. Interpretation of the significance of the parameters must be made in light of refined and realistic theories or models which account for the nature of the system to include the dominant transport mechanism, frame of reference corrections, boundary layer effects, and other relevant concepts. For engineering design purposes, the parameters can serve as phenomenological coefficients which describe the system under the given conditions without need for correction or interpretation.

A general mechanism to describe the migration of a penetrant molecule through a medium visualizes the process as a sequence of unit diffusion steps or jumps under the influence of a chemical potential (concentration) gradient by a cooperative action of the surrounding complex of molecules during which the penetrant molecule passes over a potential barrier separating one site from the next. The magnitude of the diffusion coefficient is equated as a product of a constant times the probability of a successful jump. That probability can be related to the ease of hole formation which depends on the relative mobilities of penetrant molecules and polymeric chain segments as they are affected by changes in size, shape, concentration, and interaction between components. Another major factor affecting transport is the number, size, and distribution of defect structures, such as voids, capillaries, and domain boundaries, within the polymer matrix. The inherent morphological nature of the polymer, coupled with the particular sample fabrication and processing conditions, determine the detailed defect structure.

In relatively homogeneous polymers the dependence of permeability on the anticipated controlling factors can be stated quite generally. For example, the temperature dependence of diffusion and solubility over reasonable temperature ranges can be represented by the Arhennius-type equations

$$D = D_o \exp(-E_D/RT) \quad (5)$$

$$S = S_o \exp(-\Delta H_s/RT) \quad (6)$$

where E_D is the apparent activation energy for diffusion and ΔH_s is the heat of solution. Consequently, any factor which acts to reduce the ease of hole formation for diffusion can be expected to decrease the overall rate of permeation. These effects are quite noticeable in studies of diffusion of a series of penetrants of increasing molecular size and shape since the overall transport process is extremely sensitive to the magnitude and size distribution of "holes" available per unit time and volume for diffusive jumps as determined by the inherent or modified polymer chain segmental mobilities.

The local segmental mobility or chain stiffness may be affected by chain interactions arising from hydrogen bonding, polar group interactions, or simple van der Waal's attractions. As the number of these groupings per unit chain segment length increases, the degree of interaction increases, the segmental mobility decreases, and therefore the permeation rate also decreases. These effects are especially pronounced for the case of symmetrical substitution of polar groups since the packing of adjacent chain segments is somewhat facilitated leading to more efficient interactions.

Other modifications (1-2) which serve to decrease chain segmental mobility, and therefore decrease permeation, are sufficiently high degrees of crosslinking, the presence of solid additives (fillers) onto which the polymer is strongly adsorbed, and the occurrence of crystalline domains within the polymer itself. An increase in density and crystalline content results mainly in a corresponding decrease in solubility since crystalline regions are not generally accessible for sorption. However, the concurrent permeability decrease is substantially greater, indicating that the diffusion coefficient also is decreased, presumably because of the restraining effects of crystalline regions on local chain segmental motion in adjoining non-crystalline regions and a more tortuous path through the mixture of amorphous and crystalline domains.

The local chain segmental mobility of a polymer is enhanced by the presence of an added plasticizer, resulting in a lowering of the glass transition temperature of the polymer. The permeation of solvents in a polymer is similar in that the sorbed and diffusing solvent acts to "plasticize" the polymeric system.

The net result of the much higher sorbed concentrations of good solvents in a polymer (a high K value) times the attendant plasticizing action which increases the corresponding diffusion coefficient is a marked increase in the overall permeation rate.

Typically, for low concentrations (up to about 10 percent by weight) of a sorbed penetrant, where Henry's Law is reasonably valid, the diffusion coefficient varies with concentration as:

$$D = D(c{=}o)\exp(\alpha c) \tag{7}$$

where D(c=o) is the extrapolated value of D at zero concentration and α is a characteristic parameter which can be related, for example, to the Flory-Huggins interaction parameter. For wider ranges of sorbed concentrations, better representations are obtained in terms of solvent activity, a:

$$D = D(c{=}o)\exp(\alpha' a) \tag{8}$$

This includes the regions of sorbed concentration where Henry's Law is no longer obeyed, but rather the sorption follows the Flory-Huggins equation or the related expression (2,3):

$$K = K(c{=}o)\exp(\sigma c) \tag{9}$$

Combination of Equations (8) and (9) for the case when σ approaches zero leads to Equation (7). Detailed theories have been proposed to rationalize the observed concentration dependence of diffusion, mainly in terms of free volume concepts, and to account for the phenomena of penetrant cluster formation within the polymeric matrix. We will consider some of these aspects in a later section.

In most investigations of diffusion and solution in polymers, the tacit assumption has been made that the accessible regions are structurally homogeneous so that diffusion can be considered to occur by a single activated mechanism within the continuum. Recently, however, evidence has been presented for the presence of a microporous structure in certain amorphous polymers below or near their glass temperature, and in semicrystalline polymers above their glass temperature.

The distribution of void size and shape, dependent on the manner of membrane preparation and fabrication, may range from submicrovoids of the order of unit-cell dimensions to porosities and cleavages of much greater dimensions with non-random configurations. These voids are to be distinguished from the free volume associated with liquids or amorphous solids and their magnitude is not a thermodynamic quantity. In glassy amorphous polymers as the temperature is lowered below the glass temperature, the actual total volume occupied by a polymer becomes progressively greater than the equilibrium volume of an equivalent liquid. Since segmental mobility is low, this volume difference must result in the formation of different density regions on the microscale. The less densely packed regions then correspond in effect to voids within the surrounding more densely packed matrix. This phenomenon may be even more pronounced for cellulosic polymers which exhibit very low rates of conformational rearrangement due to their inherent low segmental chain mobility.

The conditions of processing, such as casting temperature, solution composition, and subsequent annealing treatments, will have a marked effect on the microstructure of the membrane. In many cases, the resultant structural heterogeneities can be considered as voids within the terms of the above discussion. The void content will be characterized by a magnitude and size distribution which will then change with time as the membrane is subjected to more extreme environmental conditions during its use. The void distribution is directly related to the polymer chain conformation statistics.

The effect of a microporous structure on the solubility and transport properties depends on the continuity of path afforded by the distribution of microvoids and on the nature of the penetrant contained within such voids. The presence of interconnected micropores, small channels, cracks, or other flaws in polymer structure permits convection of penetrant to occur through the medium in addition to activated diffusion. Such capillary flow does not show very pronounced differences for various penetrants unless the diffusing molecule is of a dimension comparable with that of the capillary.

For the case of a homogeneous distribution of non-interconnected microvoids the overall rate of transport would be expected to increase somewhat owing to the smaller structural packing density afforded by the presence of the lower density void regions. However, when the cohesive forces between penetrant molecules are greater than the attractive forces between penetrant and polymer, the incoming penetrant tends to cluster within the polymer. With reference to the overall diffusion flux, a molecule within a cluster generally will be less mobile than an isolated free molecule owing to the additional energy required to break free from the cluster. A detailed discussion of the dependence of the diffusion flux on cluster formation as it varies with penetrant concentration, void content, time, and other factors has been presented (2,3).

A more fundamental and comprehensive approach to the general problem of diffusion in multicomponent systems is afforded by the theory of irreversible thermodynamics. The rate of flow of a substance in such a system is dependent not only on its own gradient of chemical potential (i.e., concentration gradient) but also on the gradients of chemical potential of the other components as well as external force gradients (stress, electric fields, temperature, etc.). For systems not far removed from equilibrium, this interdependence may be assumed to be linear.

The resultant cross terms have been neglected or considered negligible in almost all past investigations of diffusion. However, these terms certainly are significant in many cases, such as in so-called "active" biological transport, and therefore should be included to obtain a more complete understanding of diffusion phenomena.

Concentration Dependence of Diffusion

A major factor which may affect the performance of controlled release systems is the progressive enhancement of diffusion rates by the disruption of the polymer matrix due to swelling for one cause or another. Related effects, to either increase or diminish the rate of transport, are due to changes in the inherent mobility of the penetrant molecule caused by variations in the mode of sorption. These factors can be considered under the general concept of concentration dependence of diffusion.

As mentioned previously, the thermodynamic term ($d\ln a/d\ln\bar{c}$) in equations (1), (3), and (4) can be assessed directly from the solution theory equation which best represents the sorption isotherm for the particular system. In most cases, this term is of relatively minor significance as compared to the effects on the mobility parameter.

The mobility term, D*, in equations (1) and (3) can be further defined in terms of two concepts: a) immobilization of penetrant molecules, and b) the segmental mobility of polymer chains. The first concept involves considerations of the effects of differing modes of sorption, such as specific site solvation, chemisorption, or cluster formation, on the actual mobility of the individual penetrant molecules. The other concept considers plasticization and other effects of swelling, usually in terms of free volume treatments.

An understanding of the nature of polymer solutions suggests that one should anticipate a spectrum of penetrant molecular mobilities, $D_i(c_i)$, related to a spectrum of modes of sorption determined by the experimental time scale and the interaction energetics of various sorption sites in the system. Penetrant molecules involved in specific site sorption or in physical clusters (penetrant-rich domains below liquid nucleation size) can be considered as localized if the rate of exchange of molecules between those modes of sorption and freely diffusing species is slower than the rate of the unit diffusion process.

In the simplest case, we can consider the dual sorption mode approximation which defines the total sorbed concentration, $\bar{c}$, as composed of freely diffusing species of concentration, $\bar{c}_f$, and bound species of concentration $\bar{c}_b$. With the assumption that the bound species is totally immobilized ($D_b = 0$), equation (1) may be rewritten as:

$$J = -D_f(d\ln a_f/d\ln\bar{c}_f)(d\bar{c}_f/d\bar{c})(d\bar{c}/dc)(dc/dx) \qquad (10)$$

The experimentally determined diffusion coefficient is then:

$$D = D_f(d\ln a_f/d\ln\bar{c}_f)(d\bar{c}_f/d\bar{c}) \qquad (11)$$

The context of the assumption is such that the freely diffusing species can be considered to form an ideal solution mixture so that equation (11) can be stated as simply:

$$D = D_f(\bar{c}_f/\bar{c}) \qquad (12)$$

Thus any process which tends to localize penetrant molecules within the diffusion medium will cause $\bar{c}_f$ to be less than $\bar{c}$ and the experimentally determined value of D will be less than the "true" value D_f. This phenomenon has been extensively confirmed and the model treatments extended (4).

There have been several model relationships proposed to account for the effects of sorbed low molecular weight material to plasticize the polymer and so increase the rate of diffusion. The general method has been to estimate the probability of a successful diffusion jump in terms of either the energy required for a critical volume disturbance or free volume effects (3,5). Those based on free volume concepts have gained the widest acceptance but the energy considerations show greater promise for extended treatments to elucidate the nature of the diffusion mechanism.

In the free volume model proposed by Fujita and Kishimoto (24-26), the probability of hole formation is related to the probability of obtaining a free volume domain of a size sufficient to allow a diffusion jump (as defined for other processes by Cohen and Turnbull and by Doolittle). The diffusion coefficient is stated as

$$D^* = D(d\ln\bar{c}/d\ln a) = A_D\exp(-B_D/f) \qquad (13)$$

where A_D is a constant at a given temperature, f is the free volume fraction, and B_D is a parameter, characteristic of the system, which gives a measure of the efficiency of use of available free volume by the diffusion process.

According to the WLF equation, the temperature dependence of free volume in undiluted polymer at $T > T_g$ is

$$f(o,T) = f(o,T_g) + \alpha_2(T - T_g) \qquad (14)$$

where T_g is the glass temperature of pure (dry) polymer and α_2

is the difference between the thermal expansion coefficients above and below T_g. Provided the concentration of diluent is not too high, the concentration dependence at a given sorbed volume fraction, ϕ_1, of penetrant at a given temperature T may be given as

$$f(\phi_1,T) = f(o,T) + \beta\phi_1 = f_o + \beta\phi_1 \qquad (15)$$

where β is a parameter representing the contribution of the diluent toward increasing the free volume. β is a function of T but, to a first approximation, is independent of ϕ_1. The concentration dependence of diffusion at a given temperature is then

$$\ln[D^*/D(o)] = \beta B_D\phi_1/[f_o^2 + f_o\beta\phi_1] \qquad (16)$$

where D(o) is the value of D* at $\phi_1 = 0$. Under conditions such that $\beta\phi_1/f_o << 1$, this equation reduces to

$$\ln[D^*/D(o)] = \beta B_D\phi_1/f_o^2 \qquad (17)$$

and lnD*(and lnD) is approximately linear with ϕ_1 (corresponding to equation (7)). These relationships can represent data over ranges of concentration and swelling corresponding to those found in applications of practical membrane systems. They allow useful predictions to be made of anticipated behavior based on available material parameters.

The free volume approach to diffusion behavior also is of interest in that it brings to the forefront the correspondence between mass transfer and momentum transfer in polymeric systems (27-29). Rheological and mechanical properties of polymers, such as viscosity, creep, stress-relaxation, and dynamic-mechanical behavior, are likewise determined by the nature of the chain segmental motion processes in polymers, both in the absence and presence of a diluent. Many successful model treatments to explain and predict various relaxation processes are based on free volume concepts.

The correspondence between diffusion processes and stress relaxation processes in a series of random copolymers of isoprene and methylmethacrylate has been measured using the derived relationship, in terms of free volume as above, in the form:

$$\ln[D^*/D(o)] = (B_D/B_\eta)\ln(a_c)_o \qquad (18)$$

where:

$$(a_c)_o = \eta_o\phi_2/\eta(\phi_1)$$

η_o = viscosity(or modulus) at $\phi_1 = o$

$\eta(\phi_1)$ = viscosity at $\phi_1 = \phi_1$

The parameters B_D and B_η characterize the efficiencies by which the processes of penetrant diffusion and stress relaxation utilize the available free volume in the system. It is found that the ratio (B_D/B_η) tends to unity as the size of the penetrant molecule increases. This is in accord with the realization that for sufficiently high molecular weight penetrants, the diffusion process corresponds with that for self-diffusion of polymer segments and chains.

Since many agents in controlled release applications are of moderately high molecular weight, it seems appropriate to assess their transport behavior in analogy to the viscous flow behavior of the polymeric matrix. Thus, an appraisal of the log modulus versus time-temperature-concentration master curve gives at least qualitative indication of the behavior to be expected in a system with variations in those parameters. As time, temperature, or diluent concentration increase, the rate of diffusion (inversely related to viscosity) should increase in accord with the decrease in modulus. The decrease in modulus with added plasticizer is well known and well represented by model treatments.

A complication in prediction by the above correlation method is due to the possibility of non-uniform swelling of a polymer by a diluent. In such a case, the unswollen domains distributed through an otherwise swollen matrix would correspond in effect to a dispersed impermeable filler. If the degree of swelling is extensive, the system would resemble a porous diffusion medium. Correction for these effects can be made on the basis of model treatments derived for those cases as indicated earlier.

The permeation of large molecules in relatively non-swollen media can be treated by the realization that the differences in diffusion coefficients will be relatively small between homologous members due to the relatively small number of suitable holes or free volume domains of appropriate size for diffusion jumps. Therefore, the net flux will be determined more by the solubility level differences between penetrant species than by mobility, per se.

The solubility can be estimated by use of typical polymer solution theory expressions such as the simplified form of the Flory-Huggins equation

$$\ln a_1 = \ln\phi_1 + \phi_2 + \chi_1\phi_2^2 \tag{19}$$

The characteristic parameter χ_1 can be estimated, in turn, by the Hildebrand equation

$$\chi_1 = \bar{v}_1/RT(\delta_1 - \delta_2)^2 \tag{20}$$

The solubility parameters, δ, can be estimated by group contribution methods, heat of vaporization data, or other methods. This general approach has been used and extended to predict the release rate characteristics of steroids from polymers with considerable success (30).

Conclusion

The diffusion-solution model for understanding and predicting controlled release rates can be extended to include many other aspects and factors. Of particular interest is the strong dependence of transport behavior on polymer composition, structure, and morphology. Modifications of these system variables can be achieved by careful selection, fabrication, and post-fabrication chemical and/or physical treatments. The use of multicomponent polymer media offers advantages for enhanced and better controlled flux behavior. The development of specific polymeric formulations for particular agents and application conditions is not only desirable but also possible. The basis for that development rests, in part, on obtaining and extending our knowledge of the dependence of transport processes on the nature of the system components and their interaction with the application environment.

Literature Cited

1. Crank, J. and Park, G. S., eds. "Diffusion in Polymers", Academic Press, New York, 1968.
2. Rogers, C. E., in "Physics and Chemistry of the Organic Solid State", D. Fox, M. Labes, and A. Weissberger, eds., Vol. II, Wiley-Interscience, New York, 1965, Chap. 6.
3. Rogers, C. E. and Machin, D., CRC Critical Reviews of Macromolecular Science, (1972), 1, 245.
4. Hopfenberg, H. B., ed., "Permeability of Plastic Films and Coatings to Gases, Vapors, and Liquids", Vol. 6 of Polymer Science and Technology, Plenum Press, New York, 1974.
5. Crank, J., "The Mathematics of Diffusion", 2nd Ed., Clarendon Press, Oxford, 1975.
6. Flynn, G. L., Yalkowsky, S. H., and Roseman, T. J., J. Pharmaceutical Sci., (1974), 63, 479.
7. Tanquary, A. C. and Lacey, R. E., Eds., "Controlled Release of Biologically Active Agents", Vol. 47 of Advances in Experimental Medicine and Biology, Plenum Press, New York, 1974.
8. Cardarelli, N. F., Ed., "Controlled Release Pesticide Symposium", The University of Akron, 1974.
9. Harris, F. W., Ed., "Proceedings 1975 International Controlled Release Pesticide Symposium", Wright State University, Dayton, Ohio, 1975.
10. Williams, A., "Sustained Release Pharmaceuticals", Noyes Development Corp., Parkridge, N. J., 1969.

11. Allan, G. G., Chopra, C. S., Friedhoff, J. F., Gara, R. I., Maggi, M. W., Neogi, A. N., Roberts, S. C., and Wilkens, R. M., "Pesticides, Pollution, and Polymers", Chemtech., (1973), 3, 171.
12. Colbert, J. C., "Controlled Action Drug Forms", Noyes Data Corp., Park Ridge, N. J., 1974.
13. Cardarelli, N. F., "Concepts in Controlled Release-Emerging Pest Control Technology", Chemtech., (1975), 5, 482.
14. Baker, R. W. and Lonsdale, H. K., "Controlled Delivery-An Emerging use for Membranes", Chemtech., (1975), 5, 668.
15. Cardarelli, N. F., "Controlled Release Pesticides Formulations", CRC Press, Cleveland, Ohio, 1976.
16. Paul, D. R. and Harris, F. W., eds., "Controlled Release Polymeric Formulations", ACS Symposium Series 33, Am. Chem. Soc., Washington, D. C., 1976.
17. Chang, T. M. S., Artifical Cells, C. C. Thomas, Springfield, Ill., 1972.
18. Gutcho, M., "Capsule Technology and Microencapsulation", Noyes Data Corp., Park Ridge, N. J., 1972.
19. Vandegaer, J. E., Ed., "Microencapsulation-Processes and Applications", Plenum Press, New York, 1974.
20. Fanger, C. O., "What Good are Microcapsules", Chemtech., (1974), 4, 397.
21. Goodwin, J. T. and Somerville, G. R., "Microencapsulation by Physical Methods", Chemtech., (1974), 4, 623.
22. Chang, T. M. S., "Artificial Cells", Chemtech., (1975), 5, 80.
23. Thies, C., "Physicochemical Aspects of Microencapsulation", Polymer-Plast. Technol. Eng., (1975), 5(1), 1.
24. Fujita, H., Fortschr. Hochpolym. Forsch., (1961), 3, 1.
25. Fujita, H. and Kishimoto, A., J. Chem. Phys., (1961), 34, 393.
26. Fujita, H. and Kishimoto, A., J. Polym. Sci., (1958), 28, 547, 569.
27. Machin, D. and Rogers, C. E., J. Polym. Sci. A2, (1972), 10, 887.
28. Machin, D. and Rogers, C. E., J. Polym. Sci., Phys., (1973) 11, 1535, 1555.
29. Rogers, C. E., Semancik, J. R., and Kapur, S., Polym. Sci. Tech., (1973), 1, 297.
30. Michaels, A. S., Wong, P. S. L., Prather, R. and Gale, R. M., AlChE J., (1975), 21, 1073.

3

A Challenge for Controlled Release Pesticide Technology

PHILIP C. KEARNEY

Agricultural Environmental Quality Institute, U.S. Department of Agriculture, Beltsville, Md. 20705

Controlled release pesticide technology holds great promise for improving the efficacy of some existing pesticides and reducing the environmental problems associated with others. Previous controlled released technology has been concerned with finding the correct matrix for combining the pesticide in a form that will alter its availability to the target organism. Controlled-release formulations, which improve pesticide performance are now under investigation. Some of the greatest challenges to the new field of technology, however, may be in altering the environmental behavior of pesticides. Several environmental parameters, including volatility, photodecomposition, leaching, microbial metabolism, binding, and accumulation, determine the persistence, distribution, and indirectly the efficacy of pesticides. Laboratory and field techniques have been developed, which allow for the measurement of some of these environmental parameters affecting pesticides. These techniques offer opportunities of studying the effects of formulation on persistence and movement of pesticides.

The purpose of this paper is to challenge scientists engaged in controlled-release technology to consider some of the broader opportunities offered for improving pesticide efficacy and safety. The ability to manipulate the concentration of the toxin presented to the pest and the environment may make some older compounds more attractive commercially and may overcome some problems associated with potentially useful new compounds that otherwise might not be registered. The following discussion will center primarily on the organic herbicides, since the author's expertise is more extensive in this branch of pesticide chemistry.

Persistence

The opportunity of altering the persistence of certain herbicides seems to be one of the primary advantages of controlled-release technology. There is a group of extremely useful herbicides that unfor-

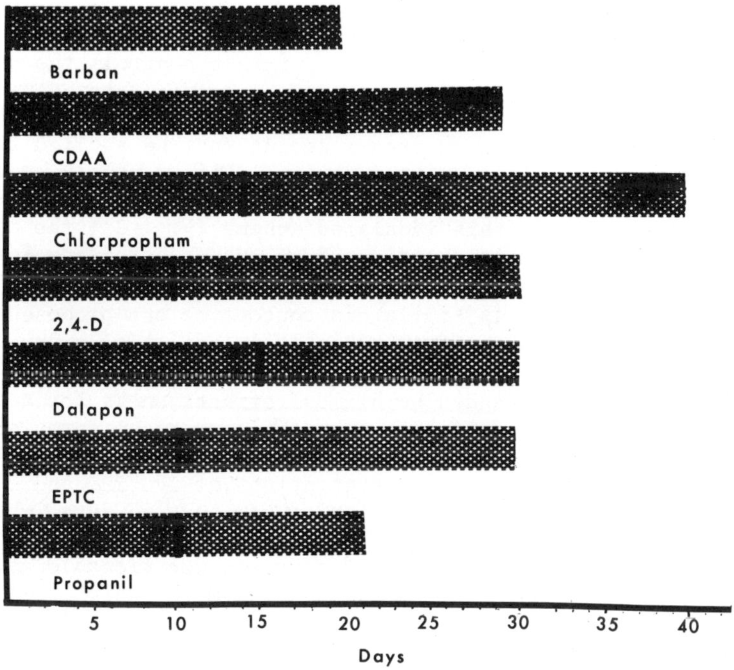

Figure 1. Persistence of seven herbicides in soil. The length of each bar represents the time required for 90% loss of the herbicide from the site of application.

tunately do not persist long enough under actual field usage to afford full-season weed control. Some of these least-persistent compounds are shown in Figure 1, where the length of the bar represents the time for 90% loss. From an environmental standpoint, these commpounds have been studied extensively and seem to offer no major problems.

The role that controlled-release technology can bring to improved weed control can be represented in a diagram recently suggested by Dawson (1976) (Fig 2). One of the factors governing herbicide selectivity is the maximum amount of herbicide tolerated by the crop plant and the minimum amount that controls the weed. Herbicides are generally applied at some economic rate between these two limits. If the herbicide degrades according to a first-order reaction rate, then an excess amount must be applied to achieve a reasonably long control period. Unfortunately, many of the short-term herbicides are dissipated before desired control level is achieved. In this idealized scheme (Fig. 2), the controlled release (CR) formation provides just enough herbicide for weed control at any one time, and the period of activity is significantly extended. Figure 2 is similar in concept to one proposed by Cowan (1973) for responses from a single injection of a drug.

Microencapsulation of chlorpropham, one of the short-lived herbicides (Fig 1), extended herbicidal effectiveness for a significantly longer period of time than the commercial formulation (Gentner and Danielson, 1976). A 4.5 kg/ha application of microencapsulated chlorpropham at concentrations of 17, 22, and 26 percent were herbicidally effective for longer than 66 days, while a similar application of the commercial formulation was completely inactive after 41 days, and its efficacy was questionable after 31 days. Volatilization is one of the mechanisms by which chlorpropham is lost from the site of application. Turner et al. (1977) compared the vapor losses of chlorpropham in a microencapsulated formulation with those in an emulsifiable concentrate under field conditions. In the first 4 hours after application, 86 g/ha of the emulsifiable and 5.3 g/ha microencapsulated chlorpropham were volatilized from the target area. Soil analysis confirmed that after 7 days, 26% of the applied emulsifiable concentrate and 51% of the microencapsulated chlorpropham remained in the target area.

A major benefit that controlled release technology can bring to weed control is to expand herbicide selectivity to additional crops. As illustrated in Figure 3, based on a suggestion by Dawson (1976), the amount of herbicide required to control weeds in crop A may injure crop B. Unfortunately, the amount of herbicide tolerated by crop B is too low to provide a sufficient period of weed control. The controlled-release formulation provides a continuous amount of herbicide at a level sufficient to control weeds but not injure either crop.

Several experimental techniques are now available for measuring the effect of controlled-release formulations on the mechanism

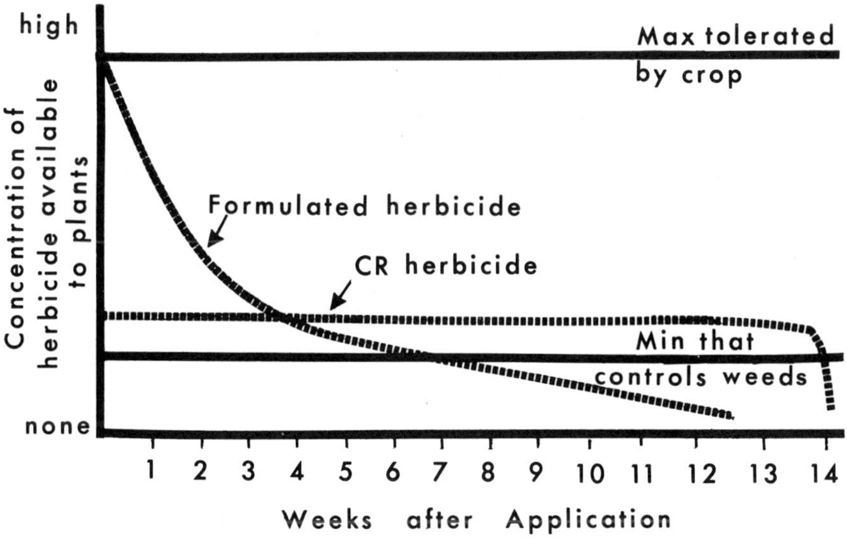

Figure 2. Degradation of formulated and controlled release (CR) herbicide as a function of time in a single-crop system

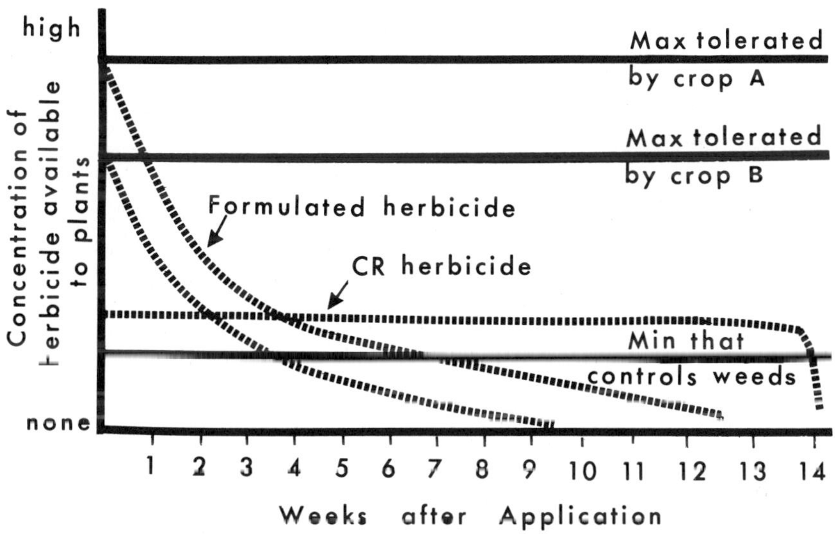

Figure 3. Degradation of formulated and controlled release (CR) herbicide as a function of time in a two-crop system

and rate of herbicide loss. Turner and Glotfelty (1977) measured volatility losses under field conditions by many polyurethane foam plugs. A simple modification of the polyurethane foam plug technique has been adopted by Kearney and Kontson (1976) to measure both volatilization and metabolic metabolism under laboratory conditions. The development of the agroecosystem by Beall et al. (1976) offers another, more elaborate, technique for analyzing various environmental components that effect a pesticide molecule in a closed system. Agroecosystems are inexpensive to construct and operate, and offer many advantages over conventional growth chambers for balance studies on pesticides. All of these systems offer scientists engaged in controlled-release technology several methods for measuring volatility, degradation, and persistence under both laboratory and field conditions.

The most challenging concept in altering herbicide persistence has been to shorten the effective life of some of the more stable compounds. To date, there is limited experimental evidence that some compounds can be rendered less persistent. Early work with the phenoxy herbicides (Audus, 1960) showed that soil induced to metabolize MCPA would also metabolize several phenoxyacetic acids supplied to it faster than would uninduced soil. This suggested that soil microbial populations would be induced to metabolize a particular class of herbicides, and more specifically a linkage in the molecule common to members of that class. In field studies, MCPA was found to degrade significantly faster in soils previously receiving five annual applications of the herbicide than in untreated soil (Fryer and Kirkland, 1970). Therefore, it may be feasible to alter the soil microbial population near a soil-applied herbicide to accelerate its metabolism.

Loos and Kearney (1977) have attempted to alter the soil microbial environment by providing degradable substrates which structurally resemble atrazine. Previous research on atrazine degradation reveals that there are two major types of cleavage: chemical replacement of the chlorine in the 2-position with a hydroxyl group and microbial dealkylation of the ethyl group (Esser et al., 1976). In the experiments of Loos and Kearney (1977), several compounds containing carbon nitrogen bonds were applied to soils to accelerate dealkylation. These compounds included ammelide, ammeline, cyanuric acid, N-ethylammelide, N-ethylammeline, urea, biuret, and quanidine. To date, these experiments have only met with limited success.

Whether controlled-release technology could provide a vehicle for combining the herbicide and accelerator compound remains to be tested. The goal of being able to predict and modify the time of effectiveness of persistent herbicides is an exciting challenge that may yet be possible to achieve.

Movement

As discussed in the previous section, microencapsulation retarded the volatilization of CIPC and, thereby, extended its effectiveness under field conditions. Another form of movement that can reduce a herbicide's effectiveness is vertical leaching into the soil profile. For many preemergence herbicides, the compound must remain in the germination zone of the weed seedling to be effective. Metribuzin is a promising herbicide for weed control in soybeans and several other crops. The compound is somewhat water soluble and, under certain conditions, extensive vertical movement has been observed. If this movement can be controlled, then much better weed control is obtained. Recently, Savage and McCormick (1977) combined metribuzin in a polymer system, which restricted leaching and significantly improved weed control.

Several simple and sophisticated techniques are available for measuring leaching of herbicides in soils. Helling (1971) devised a soil thin-layer system, which allows for a rapid, simple method of measuring leaching. Herbicide mobility can be detected by using 14C-labeled compounds, followed by autoradiography on thicker plates; thus, nonlabeled pesticides have been visualized using bioassay organisms. Savage and McCormick (1977) used soil thin-layer mobility studies to demonstrate the slow release of metribuzin. More complex column procedures are also available for determining the leachability of particular herbicides.

New Challenges

While the most promising challenges for controlled release technology is altering pesticide persistence and movement, there may be other environmental parameters that can be modified or altered by formulation. Pesticide binding to physical and biological surfaces may be influenced by formulation. The full significance of binding is not completely understood at this time, although Kearney (1976) has discussed two aspects of pesticide binding to soils. Bound residues may be beneficial as a decontamination mechanism for inactivating pesticides in soils or undesirable as potential storage sites for subsequent release of the pesticides back into the environment. When the full implication of the beneficial or adverse effects of pesticide binding are understood, controlled release technology may provide formulations that enhance or deter binding. The carrier could preferentially interact with the binding surface to modify the nature of attachment of the pesticide. Several methods are available for measuring bound residues (Kaufman et al., 1976) and these may provide information on the effect of various formulations on the extent and strength of binding.

As controlled release pesticide technology continues to expand in the field of pesticide chemistry, new opportunities will arise for solving some of the environmental problems associated with expanded pesticide usage. One of the greatest challenges to improving controlled release technology is to develop and utilize reasonable model systems for measuring volatility, photodecomposition, metabolism, and other parameters. These simple systems offer the most reasonable approach to rapidly achieving new advances in controlled-release technology.

Literature Cited

1. Andus, L. J. in Herbicides and the Soil (E. K. Woodford and G. R. Sager, eds.), Blackwell, Oxford pp 1-19 (1960).
2. Beall, M. L., Jr., Nash, R. G., Kearney, P. C., Proc. Conf. Environ. Modeling Simulation EPA 600/9-76-016 (1976).
3. Cowan, D. R., Introduction to Controlled Release of Biologically Active Agents, Edited by A. C. Tanquary 2nd; R. E. Lacy, Plenum Press pp 1-13 (1973).
4. Dawson, J. H., Personal Communication (1976).
5. Esser, H. O., Dupuis, G., Ebert, E., Vogel, C., Marco, G. J., s-Triazines in Herbicides: Chemistry, Degradation and Mode of Action (P. C. Kearney and D. D. Kaufman, eds.) Vol. 1, pp 129-208, 2 ed., Marcel Dekker, Inc., New York (1975).
6. Fryer, J. D., Kirkland, K., Weed Res. 10, 133 (1970).
7. Gentner, W. A., Danielson, L. L., Proc. 1976 Controlled Release Pestic. Symp. 7, 27, Akron, Ohio (1976).
8. Helling, C. S., Soil Sci. Soc. Am. Proc. 35, 737 (1971).
9. Kaufman, D. D., Still, G. G., Paulson, G. D., Bandal, S. K., Bound and Conjugated Pesticide Residues. ACS Symp. Ser. 29, 396 pp. (1976).
10. Kearney, P. C., Summary of Soil Bound Residue Discussion Session in Bound and Conjugated Pesticide Residues (D. D. Kaufman, G. G. Still, G. D. Paulson and S. K. Bandal, eds.). ACS Symp. Ser. 29, 378-382 (1976).
11. Kearney, P. C., Kontson, A., J. Agric. Food Chem. 24, 424 (1976).
12. Savage, K. E., McCormick, C. L., Proc. Southern Weed Sci. Soc., Dallas, Texas (1977).
13. Turner, B. C., Glotfelty, D. E., Anal. Chem. 49, 7 (1977).
14. Turner, B. C., Glotfelty, D. E., Taylor, A. W. and Watson, D. R., 173rd Natl. Mtg. Amer. Chem. Soc. (Abstr.) #8, New Orleans, La. (1977).

4

Environmental Aspects of Controlled Release Pesticide Formulations

GUNTER ZWEIG

Environmental Protection Agency, Office of Pesticide Programs, Washington, D.C. 20460

During the past 10 years many persistent pesticides (e.g. chlorinated hydrocarbons) have been phased out because of environmental and toxicological problems. In their place, less persistent, but sometimes more acutely toxic pesticides have been substituted and created other problems: (a) greater chances for accidental, high exposure to operators and farm workers; and (b) a need for multiple applications because of lower persistence. Controlled release (CR) formulations of these pesticides appear to offer an ideal solution to these problems. To cite another consideration, the insect growth regulator methoprene, for example, is so unstable in the aquatic environment that its practical application could only be effected as a controlled release formulation. Newly developed pesticides may never reach the market unless they can be stablized long enough to effect control through controlled-release formulations. Economic and environmental advantages might also be gained by the release of constant but lower concentrations of toxicants than may be possible with conventional type formulations.

The technology of microencapsulation and other controlled release systems, as will be discussed during this Symposium, have been developed to the point of making controlled release pesticide formulations a reality. Yet, there appears to be no satisfactory explanation why this field has not advanced more rapidly. One popular explanation might be that Government regulations for toxicological and environmental testing have become so cumbersome that they discourage further development of these formulations. In this paper, some personal reflections may help to alleviate these concerns, and it may become apparent that the proposed tests are probably no more stringent than those required for conventional pesticide formulations.

Asterisked terms throughout this paper indicate trademark products.

Mention of trade names or commercial products does not constitute endorsement or recommendation for use by the U.S. Environmental Protection Agency.

Feasible CR Pesticide Formulations

Although the number of commercial controlled-release pesticide products on the market may be few compared to the more than 30,000 other registered products, it appears feasible that all classes of pesticide chemicals are amenable to formulation as controlled-release products. In a number of cases, as in the case of methoprene, the CR formulation is the method of choice and enhances the efficacy of the pesticide, albeit, makes it feasible to be used as an effective pest control agent. Table I is a list of these pesticide classes followed by a few words of explanation.

TABLE I

CLASSES OF PESTICIDES FORMULATED AS CONTROLLED-RELEASE PRODUCTS

Anti-Foulants	Rodenticides
Molluscicides	Nematicides
Insecticides	Algicides
Herbicides	Predator Control Devices
Fungicides	Repellents

Anti-foulants. Anti-fouling paints are composed of a toxicant, for example, cuprous oxide which is held within a polymeric vehicle such as polyacrylate, polyamide, polyester, chlorinated polyisoprene, polyurethane, etc. Other toxicants that have been successfully incorporated into anti-foulant paints include organotin compounds (e.g., tributyl tin) and organoleads (e.g., triphenyl lead). These anti-fouling coatings have been shown to be biologically efficacious and long lasting (up to 9 years) (1). The unresolved environmental problems with these products are (a) the possible long-term effect on aquatic organisms of low concentrations of toxicants, and (b) the characterization of the released material which may have undergone chemical or biological changes during its release.

Molluscicides. Molluscicides are used to control snails and slugs and are extremely important in tropical areas where a major disease, Schistosomiasis, is transmitted by members of the *Schistosoma* snail family inhabiting rivers, streams and lakes. N.F. Cardarelli, Professor of Chemistry, University of Akron, Ohio, has been a pioneer in the development of CR molluscicides. Tributyltin oxide (TBTO) and tributyltin fluoride, niclosamide (ethanolamine salt of 2,5-dichloro-4'-nitrosalicylanilide), and copper sulfate have been incorporated into various elastomeric materials. The toxicants are released over a period of many months following immersion into infected waters. Although the tin compounds are toxic to fish, when used as CR formulations, however, the adverse effect on fish appears minimal. Most vascular species of plants are unaffected by tributyltin oxide, although some adverse effects on algae have been observed. Other nontarget aquatic organisms appear to be tolerant to TBTO at the concentration of the CR formulations. The environmental fate of organotins is not fully understood, but tin does not seem to bioaccumulate in higher organisms and, as a matter of fact, is an essential trace element in mammalian nutrition.

Another CR technique for snail control is the use of CR baits. In this technique, the toxicant [niclosamide or trifenmorph (N-tritylmorpholine)] and an attractant are incorporated into an insoluble binding matrix (e.g., polyacrylates cross-linked with Zn^{++} or Ca^{++}). Snails are attracted by a genus-specific attractant and ingest the polymers containing the toxicant.

The use of CR molluscicides, although of minor importance in the United States, illustrates that a toxicant can be used at lower concentrations than those required by direct application and provides greater environmental safety.

Insecticides. In this category are included (a) conventional target insecticides and insect growth regulators which are formulated to produce controlled release, and (b) pheromones and other attractants which are incorporated into baits containing conventional insecticides for the kill. One of the first types of a commercial CR formulation is Penncap-M*, microencapsulated methyl parathion. The microencapsulation process is based on forming a polycondensation polymer shell (cross-linked polyamide) around the material to be encapsulated.

The insect growth regulator methoprene is incorporated into a polyurethane foam providing some degree of protection from environmental degradation. This product is sold commercially as Altsosid SR-10*.

Chlorpyrifos (1A) has been incorporated into polyvinyl chloride, polyurethane foam, and polyamide and provides excellent control of mosquito larvae over a 22 to 24-week period, as compared with 1 to 2 weeks using chlorpyrifos emulsion (2). Even longer control was effected with polyethylene or polyvinyl chloride CR pellets (3).

Encapsulated Rabon* [(Gardona* -- 2-chloro-1-(2,4,5-trichlorophenyl)vinyl dimethylphosphate] has been shown to provide larval feed-through control in the manure of poultry and cattle (4, 5).

The second category of CR insect control agents are pheromones and attractants which have been reviewed recently (6). For example, disparlure has been formulated into gelatin capsules (7) or laminated plastic dispensers (8, 9); grandlure has been formulated into laminated plastics (10); and encapsulated trimedlure has been combined with methyl parathion or malathion (11). All of these formulations have the advantage of prolonging the life of the environmentally labile and volatile pheromones.

At this time, pheromones have been identified for at least 40 economically important insect species (8), and a larger number of pheromone/toxicant or pheromone/trap systems may be expected to be developed on a commercial scale in the future.

Another type of CR insecticide formulation is represented by an anti-cockroach paint containing chlorpyrifos (12) and the Hercon* plastic insecticide dispenser incorporating chlorpyrifos, Baygon* (o-isopropoxyphenyl N-methyl carbamate), or diazinon [O,O-diethyl O-(2-isopropyl-6-methyl-4-pyrimidinyl) phosphorothioate] in a 3-layer laminated polyvinyl construction (13). DDVP (dichlorvos -- 2,2-dichlorovinyl dimethylphosphate), widely used as a CR formulation under the trade name of No-Pest* strip, is incorporated into polyvinyl chloride and montan wax. The chitin-synthesis inhibitor dimilin [1-(4-chlorophenyl)-3-(2,6-difluorobenzoyl)urea] has been experimentally incorporated into castor wax and a silicate to produce a CR formulation (14). Castor wax hydrolyzes to ricinoleic acid and glycerol with no apparent environmental consequences.

Herbicides. CR formulations of herbicides may be classified as aquatic/plastic, aquatic/elastomeric, and agricultural. Aquatic herbicides (phenoxy esters, endothall, dichlobenil) have been incorporated into polyamide, polyvinyl (15, 16), and polyethylene resin matrices (17) to provide long-term control of Eurasian watermilfoil (18). Long-term aquatic weed control is clearly possible by herbicide release from plastic matrices (19).

Another experimental approach has been to incorporate hydrolyzable phenoxy herbicide moieties into a polymerized vinyl polymer (20, 21). Other CR materials which have been tested include rubber-based compounds as sinking pellets slowly releasing the herbicide (22, 23) with no detectable fish toxicity (18). During this work the phenomenon of chronicity was discovered, which will be discussed in greater detail later in the paper.

Although the use of aquatic herbicides as controlled release formulations may receive wider acceptance, there are relatively few CR formulated commercial agricultural herbicides.

Fungicides. Fungicidal resins for paints can be made by the polycondensation of glycol, chlorophenol ester, and benzene carboxylic acid. Seed protection can be afforded by the use of CR formulations of fungicides added to rubber latex or as an encapsulated material, e.g., Benlate*, for use on onion seeds.

Rodenticides. Encapsulation of anticoagulants appears to enhance bait acceptance (24), presumably masking the bitter taste of, for example, norbormide (25). However, although encapsulation improves rodent ingestion of the anticoagulant, it does not improve the efficacy (26) possibly because of the competition between detoxication and slower release.

Nematicides. Ethoprop (O-ethyl S,S-dipropyl phosphorodithioate), incorporated into natural rubber and an ethylene-propylenediene terpolymer (27), has been shown to have an effective release of three months. Dibromodichloropropane (DBCP) has been encapsulated with a water-sensitive, biodegradable wall material (27A); this formulation may persist during dry periods until sufficient soil moisture ruptures the capsule membrane. The basic problem of processing nematicides by press cures of elastomers or hot melt extrusion of plastics is the low boiling point of most fumigant-nematicides.

Algicides. Most copper salts have a short life in water and must be applied periodically to control the growth of algae. Thus, CR formulations of Cu^{++} ions would be highly desirable. Copper sulfate has been incorporated into a microporous polymer (Envirocap*). Another CR formulation, Incracide E-51* granules, has been shown effective against blue-green algae for as long a period as 54 days after application. No published information on the composition of these CR matrices is available (28). Experimental copper releasing thermoplastic materials have been shown to release the metal ion for several months (29, 30, 31). Increasing effort in this field should yield practical algal control methods by CR technology.

Predator Control Devices. A method that might be included in this brief survey of CR pesticide formulation is the cyanide collar attached to a sacrificial lamb, which, upon attack by a coyote, is punctured and releases the deadly poison. Many objections have been raised by conservationists and members of humane societies that this type of predatory control constitutes a singularly cruel method, and EPA has made no decision at this time to allow the use of these devices.

Repellents. Diethyl-m-toluamide (DEET) can be incorporated into sprayable polymeric materials (32) like polyacrylics and polyurethane (unpublished data by N.F. Cardarelli). These formulations have been shown to release DEET on window screens for several months, while DEET alone is rapidly degraded in sunlight.

Specific Products

Table II lists some of the CR pesticide formulations which have been registered by the EPA and are commercially available. In the study funded by EPA and recently completed (EPA Contract No. 68 01 1922), Cardarelli and Walker found references in the open, patent, and company literature of 141 pesticide chemicals which are practical or have been tried as CR formulations. Thus, this list in Table II seems limited, and it is expected that additional CR products will be on the market in the future.

TABLE II

CONTROLLED RELEASE PESTICIDES

Product	Pesticide Action
Altosid*	Juvenile Hormone Mimic
Biomet*	Molluscicide
CAP-CYC*	Plant Growth Regulator
CBL-9B	Molluscide
Herbicide 14 ACE-B1	Herbicide
Hercon* roach tape	Insecticide
	Molluscide
Incracide* E-51	Algicide
	Herbicide
Killmaster*	Insecticide
Nofoul*	Anti-foulant
No-Pest* Strip	Insecticide
Penncap-M*	Insecticide
Staph-Chek*	Bacteriostat

Altosid* is the CR formulation of the insect growth regulator methoprene.

Biomet* is an organotin molluscicide.

CAP-CYC* is 3M's encapsulated chlormequat (2-chloroethyltrimethylammonium chloride), a plant growth regulator. The composition of the encapsulant and additives are not public information.

CBL-9B is a natural rubber matrix containing tributyltin fluoride as active molluscicide.

Herbicide 14 ACE-B1 is the 2,4-D butoxyethanol ester formulated with natural rubber; this has been prepared as floating or sinking pellets and suspending strands, depending on the nature of the vulcanized elastomers.

Hercon* roach tape utilizes the Hercon dispenser constructed from laminar strips containing an insecticide in a plastic reservoir. Hercon* roach tape containing Baygon* is effective as a stationary insecticide dispenser especially useful against cockroaches around human habitation.

Incracide* E-51 is a terpolymer CR formulation of copper sulfate intended as a molluscicide, algicide, and selective herbicide.

Killmaster* is a paintable or sprayable CR formulation containing chlorpyrifos.

Nofoul* is an anti-fouling rubber, the principle of which rests on diffusion-dissolution. The ingredients are proprietary information.

No-Pest* Strip is probably the best known CR formulation and is composed of dichlorvos in a stabilized polyvinyl chloride base.

Penncap-M* is a widely used CR insecticide and is polyamide-encapsulated methyl parathion. At 25%-cross linkage of the polymer wall, the efficacy of Penncap-M* against the bollworm and bollweevil was extended from one day to about 10 days when compared with conventional emulsifiable concentrate (EC) formulations (33). Comparative toxicity data indicate that Penncap-M* is approximately 50 times less toxic to rabbits by skin absorption, 8 to 10 times less toxic to white mice, and 4 to 7 times less toxic to rats by ingestion than the corresponding EC formulation. An unexpected hazard of Penncap-M* to the bee population has been discovered recently (34). The microcapsules, which are approximately the same size as pollen grains, adhere to the bee as it flies from sprayed flowers and returns the "pollen" to the hive where it contaminates the whole colony.

Staph-Chek* is a bacteriostatic fabric used in hospitals. Organotin or another bacteriocide(stat) is incorporated into PVC film which is laminated on a fabric base.

Other CR pesticide products and commercial release systems are shown in Table III.

TABLE III

CONTROLLED RELEASE PRODUCTS

Polyethylene/chlorpyrifos Blend 3714
Conrel*
Hercon* Dispenser
Microcapsule Dispenser
Poroplastic*
Sustrelle*

Polyethylene - chlorpyrifos is a CR mosquito larvicide developed by the U.S. Army Environmental Hygiene Agency; registration by the EPA has been applied for.

Conrel* is a trademark for a wide range of precision hollow fiber systems, especially suitable for volatile pesticides and pheromones. Controlled vapor release rates can be achieved by tailoring the fibers to specific diameters and lengths.

The Hercon* Dispenser has been described previously.

Microcapsule Dispenser. No information is available about the composition of the Microcapsule Dispenser produced by Controlled Release Chemical Corporation, Santa Fe, N. Mex. The dispenser is useful for releasing pheromones and insecticides.

Poroplastic* (sheets) and Sustrelle* are trade names for gelled cellulose triacetate. The cost of these materials is relatively high to make them practical for use at this time, but in principle, they should function as a sustained and controlled release system.

Environmental Impact of Polymers

Before considering the environmental impact of CR pesticide formulations, it is important to briefly review the polymeric materials, or the so-called "inerts," which make up the bulk of these types of formulations. Table IV is a list of significant polymers that were chosen for closer investigation.

TABLE IV

CONTROLLED RELEASE MATERIALS

Rubber	Polyethylene
Natural	Polyvinyl Chloride
Synthetic	Chloroprene Polymer
Ethylene - Propylene Polymer	Polyurethanes
Cellulosic Materials	Cis Polybutadiene
Polyisobutylene - Butyl Rubber	Acetal Copolymer
Styrene - Butadiene Copolymer	Others:
Polyacrylonitriles	Silicon Rubber
Polyacrylates	Polyacrylamides
Polyesters	Hydrin Rubber
Polyamides	Microporous Plastic Sheet

A direct quotation by Cardarelli and Walker in their final report to the EPA on the Development of Registration Criteria for CR Pesticide Formulations, sums up their views on the environmental impact from the use of CR pesticide products:

> "It should be recognized that the polymeric material must degrade in some fashion before there can be any environmental impact in the chemical, biochemical or biological sense. With reference to soil or the beds of watercourses, it is conceivable, though barely, that the addition of a polymer to the ambient environment will result in physical changes. It is well known that the application of an inert material to soil aids in aeration. Thus, a non-

degraded polymer plowed into soil will enhance soil aeration. Since the authors cannot visualize more than a few hundred pounds per acre of a given polymer being applied annually (a few pounds per acre being much more likely), and since the weight of an acre-foot of soil is in excess of a million pounds, the environmental impact after dilution would appear to be nil. If polymers for use in controlled release were completely inert - or their degradation rate was measured in geologic time - as occurs with glass, the cumulative aspect would be a matter of concern. However, all organic polymers degrade upon exposure to outdoor environment, and with few exceptions their nature is completely obliterated after a number of decades."

Degradation of polymers occurs by one or all of the following mechanisms:

1. Solar radiation (especially ultraviolet)
2. Heat
3. Hydrolysis
4. Oxidation (oxygen or ozone)
5. Biological degradation

In conventional polymer technology, it is usually the intent to prevent environmental degradation by modifying the polymeric structure or to add stabilizers. There appears ample literature on the degradation of polymers in order to improve the final product. A number of plastics and polymers appear as food-contact materials in packaging or closures and have been exempted from a tolerance by the EPA under section 40 CFR 180.1001. Yet it is prudent to raise questions on the environmental impact, especially in light of the current interest on the so-called "inerts" in pesticide products.

Natural Rubber degrades rapidly upon environmental exposure through microbial, oxidative, and photochemical action. Normally, anti-oxidants and preservatives are added to rubber to extend its life, but rubber formulations can be tailored to increase degradation, if this is desired. Chlorinated natural rubber, now in use in anti fouling coatings, is highly resistant to biological attack but may be toxic to microorganisms (Unpublished observations, N.F. Cardarelli).

Ethylene Propylene Polymers show relatively little degradation caused by heat, humidity or uv-radiation, ozone attack, and oxidation.

Cellulosic Materials generally degrade under environmental conditions when exposed to the atmosphere and sunlight. Bacterial decay in loose, moist soil is extremely rapid. Cellulose triacetate has been cleared for food contact usage. Carboxymethylcelluloses are used in foods as gellants and thickeners and are essentially nontoxic to man.

Polyisobutylene and Butyl Rubber. Compounded butyl rubber materials are highly resistant to moisture and fairly resistant to oxidation. Addition of peroxides, however, will accelerate their breakdown. The degree of environmental impact depends on the curing agent (e.g., sulfur or lead peroxide). Generally speaking, butyl rubber degradation by environmental factors appears to proceed very slowly. No information has been found on environmental breakdown products.

Styrene - Butadiene Copolymers are very susceptible to attack by oxygen, ozone, and uv-radiation. Compared to natural rubber, these compounds exhibit a greater resistance to bacterial attack. Identification of metabolism or breakdown products has not been found in the literature surveyed.

Polyacrylonitriles tend to be resistant to microbial degradation, but ozone degrades these materials rapidly.

Polyacrylates. Carboxylated acrylic systems such as Carboset* are readily degraded by microorganisms, especially fungi. Carboset* polymers are ingested by molluscs, insects, and probably nematodes (personal observation, N.F. Cardarelli). Carboset* 514 has been exempted by EPA from the requirements of a tolerance when used in agriculture (CFR 40 Sect. 180.1001). No information is available on the toxicity of Carboset* to fish or plants or any other segment of the biota; no environmental fate studies have been conducted by the manufacturer.

Polyesters are known for their resistance to chemical and radiation-induced degradation. Breakdown products at elevated temperatures include allyl alcohol, acetaldehyde, carbon dioxide, water, formic and acetic acids. No information on possible biodegradation was found.

Polyamides degrade under the influence of heat and radiation to simple hydrocarbons and cyclopentanone. Under ambient environmental conditions, however, the degradation of Nylon microcapsules is expected to be very slow. No environmental studies were found in this survey. Exemption has been granted by the EPA under CFR 40 Sect. 180.1001.

Polyethylene (PE). Polyethylene, chlorinated- and chlorosulfonated PE's have been used for CR matrices (e.g., chlorpyrifos/PE, Table III) and are generally resistant to environmental degradation and microbial attack.

Polyvinyl Chloride is degraded at different rates depending on the plasticizer used: phthalate and phosphate plasticizers -- stable; adipate, azelate, and sebacate plasticizers -- susceptible to degradation. The possibility of vinyl chloride monomer present in the plastic or as a degradation product must be investigated.

Chloroprene polymers are highly resistant to microbial attack (35, 36).

Polyurethanes are especially prone to fungal and bacterial attack (35) but are resistant to chemical degradation.

Cis Polybutadiene is thermally stable, and although environmental studies were not found in this survey, it is suspected that these polymers behave similarly to natural rubber.

Acetal Copolymers, used in the Conrel* delivery system (Table III), may degrade to formaldehyde and ethylene oxide in soil and water, although no hard data could be found to verify this hypothesis.

Other Materials. Although silicone rubber is not presently used in CR pesticide formulations, it has found usage in CR drug delivery systems and thus may find future applications in pesticide products. Silicones are recognized as nontoxic and extremely inert to biological attack.

Polyacrylamides are not presently used for pesticide formulations; these materials degrade slowly under the influence of heat, and it is anticipated that they will gradually depolymerize to ammonia or ammonium ions depending on pH. Hydrin rubber represents another CR matrix for pesticides; it is the homopolymer of epichlorohydrin. Hydrin rubber is stable to heat and ozone but might be susceptible to microbial attack. The Microporous Plastic Sheet* is made of silica modified PVC or vinyl chloride-vinyl acetate copolymers. It is a likely candidate for CR formulations, but little is known about its environmental behavior.

Polymer - Additives

Space does not permit extensive discussion of the nature and environmental impact of polymer additives. These additives are a variety of plasticizers, antioxidants, release regulators, etc. Many of these compounds are exempt from tolerance (CFR 40, Sect. 180.1001), although some, like the phthalates, have been shown to exhibit toxicological and environmental problems. However, one would have to assess their escape from the CR system to evaluate possible environmental and human exposure. For a more complete description of these additives and toxicological evaluation, the reader is referred to the EPA Report on CR Pesticide Formulations (EPA Contract No. 68-01-1922).

Toxicological and Environmental Testing

Generally speaking, CR formulations of pesticides and the conventional emulsifiable concentrate or wettable powder formulations are not considered different entities under present pesticide laws and regulations. The pesticide law (FIFRA as amended in 1972 and 1975) addresses itself to "pesticides" and its intent is to regulate each of the approximately 30,000 pesticide products. The Guidelines for Registering Pesticides in the United States, which are presently undergoing final revisions before publication, clearly distinguish between the "technical chemical," which pesticide scientists have always considered to be synonomous with "pesticide," and "pesticide formulations," which the legislators have termed "pesticides". It is doubtful that any regulations now or in the future will require detailed toxicological and environmental testing for each pesticide formulation.

Detailed toxicological and environmental tests will have to be performed on the technical material (or so-called "active ingredient"), although some attention will be directed towards the so-called "inert" ingredients, which have been discussed in detail above for controlled-release formulations. It appears that most matrices so far utilized for CR pesticide formulations may be covered by CFR 40 Section 180.1001 (exempt category), although this decision must be made on each individual basis.

The crux of the unresolved question might be phrased like this: Does the active ingredient placed into a plastic capsule behave differently toxicologically than if it were formulated more conventionally as an emulsifiable concentrate or a dust?

Toxicological Testing. Detailed discussions on this topic will be covered in the chapter by J. Doull. The best example of lower toxicity, which one would generally expect from a controlled- or slow-release formulation, is the case of Penncap-M* compared to methyl parathion emulsifiable concentrate. As discussed above, the dermal and oral toxicity of the CR formulation was considerably lower than that of the emulsifiable concentrate (33). Table V is a listing of the major toxicological tests now required by the EPA for registration purposes.

TABLE V

MAJOR TOXICOLOGICAL TESTS FOR REGISTRATION OF PESTICIDES

Acute Oral	Acute Dermal
Subacute Oral	Subacute Dermal
Chronic (incl. cancer)	Acute Inhalation
Eye Irritation	Teratogenicity
Dermal Irritation	Mutagenicity

If the complete tests have been performed on the pesticide chemical itself, it appears reasonable that only the acute tests may be required for the CR product.

Environmental Testing. As has been discussed before, the lack of knowledge about the environmental fate of CR matrices makes it difficult to reach a decision on which environmental tests should be required. Furthermore, the mechanism of controlled release of small concentrations of a toxicant over an extended period of time may present environmental problems that cannot be predicted. Two problems, those of "chronicity" and "resistance" have been identified and will be discussed below. Therefore, it is only possible to summarize environmental test requirements and for each test to pose the question: "Is it reasonable to assume that the CR formulation behaves differently than, for example, an EC formulation?" Table VI is a summary of the required environmental tests proposed in the EPA Guidelines for Registering Pesticides soon to be published.

TABLE VI

ENVIRONMENTAL TESTS

Hydrolysis	Field dissipation Terrestrial Aquatic Forest
Photolysis	
Metabolism Aerobic soil Anaerobic soil Aerobic aquatic Anaerobic aquatic Microbial on pesticides on microbes activated sludge	Accumulation Rotational crops Fish accumulation Aquatic noncrop uses Reentry Dislodgeable residues Volatility Photodegradation
Mobility Leaching Volatility Adsorption/desorption Water dispersal	Procedures for disposal and storage

"Chronicity" Phenomenon. Chronic intoxication requires much less of the control agent than that necessary to produce acute effects. As the concentration of the agent is decreased, the time to effect lethality does not increase linearly. This phenomenon has been termed "chronicity" by Cardarelli (37) and has been demonstrated with a number of CR formulations of phenoxy herbicides, diquat, and dichlobenil to control aquatic weeds like water lettuce, Eurasian watermilfoil, Elodea, Southern naiad, and water hyacynth. "Chronicity" has also been demonstrated with antifouling agents, incorporated into certain rubbery materials, and molluscicides. The butoxyethanol ester of 2,4-D, compounded into natural rubber, has been shown to yield effective control concentrations for over 18 months. From the point of view of efficacy, the "chronicity" phenomenon may be advantageous. On the other hand, whether the phenomenon poses an environmental hazard, for example to fish, remains to be resolved. An example of "chronicity" is illustrated in Table VII, which shows the extended control of watermilfoil by diquat over a 32-day period at different concentrations of diquat tested (38).

TABLE VII

THE CONTROL OF EURASIAN WATERMILFOIL BY DIFFERENT CONCENTRATIONS OF DIQUAT

CONCN. OF DIQUAT (PPM)	LT_{99} [a] (Days)
1.0	11
0.1	19
0.01	16
0.001	32

[a] Time which 99% control is effected

The Resistance Problem. The use of controlled-release pesticides (larvicides) may well enhance the resistance problem. Sublethal dosages of insecticides tend to lead to the development of more resistant populations. Since controlled release larvicides will be conceptually used in very low concentrations, and long-term release will be achieved for cost effectiveness, considerable sublethal dosing can be expected. This effect results in many generations of the same species in the same locale exposed to the action of the larvicide. The problem of enhanced tolerance (or resistance) through the use of controlled methods has yet to be investigated.

Summary

A survey of the types of controlled-release formulations of different classes of pesticides has been presented. Some CR pesticide formulations have become commercial products, while others are still experimental and feasible but have not been tested. A discussion of the various CR matrices has shown that the environmental fate of many inerts is unknown and should be studied before they are introduced into the environment. At the present state of knowledge there do not seem to be serious environmental problems except for possible resistance and toxicity to nontarget populations of beneficial insects.

Acknowledgements

This paper is largely based on a study funded by EPA, Contract No. 68-01-1922, Development of Registration Criteria for Controlled Release Pesticides, and special thanks are due to the authors of this report, N.F. Cardarelli, K.E. Walker, and M. Beroza.

General References

Cardarelli, N.F. Controlled Release Pesticide Formulations. CRC Press, Cleveland, Ohio, 210 pp. (1976).

Proc. Controlled Release Pesticide Symposium, Univ. of Akron, Ohio. (1974, 1976).

Proc. Controlled Release Pesticide Symposium, Wright State Univ., Dayton, O. (1975).

Literature Cited

1. Wuerzer, D.R., Senderling, R.L., and Cardarelli, N.F. Rubber World, (Nov. 1967) 157 (2), 77.

1A. Nelson, L.L., Barnes, W.W., Harris, F.W. and Lawson, M.A., J. Econ. Entomol. (1970) 63, 1870.

2. Miller, T.A., Nelson, L.L., Young, W.W., Roberts, L.W., Roberts, D.R. and Wilkinson, R.N., Mosq. News, (1973) 33 148.

3. Nelson, L.L., Miller, T.A., Whitlaw, J.T., Young, W.W., and Lawson, M.A., Mosq. News, (1973) 33, 403.

4. Wasti, S.S., Shaw, F.R. and Smith, C.T., J. Econ. Entomol. (1970) 63, 1355.

5. Miller, R.W., Drazek, P.A., Martin, M.S. and Gordon, C.H., Rep. No. 169, Ann. Mtng. Amer. Dairy Sci. Assoc., Gainesville, Fla. DCRB 70-8, (June 1970).

6. Inscoe, M.N. and Beroza, M. in Pest Management with Insect Sex Attractants, (pp. 145-181), M. Beroza, ed., ACS Symposium Series 23, Amer., Chem. Soc., Wash., D.C. (1976).

7. Cameron, E.A., Schwalbe, C.P., Stevens, L.J. and Beroza, M., J. Econ. Entomol., (1975) 68, 158.

8. Bierl, B.A. and DeVilbiss, D., Proc. Controlled Release Pesticide Symp., 230, Wright State University, Dayton, OH, (September 8-10, 1975).

9. Beroza, M., Paszek, E.C., DeVilbiss, D., Bierl, B.A. and Tardif, J.G.R., Environ. Entomol., (1975) 4, 712.

10. Hardee, D.C., McKibben, G.H. and Huddleston, P.M., J. Econ. Entomol., (1975) 68, 477.

11. Keiser, I., Kobayashi, R.M. and Harris, E.J., Proc. Controlled Release Pesticide Symp., 264, Wright State University, Dayton, OH, (September 8-10, 1975).
12. Olton, G.S., Proc. Controlled Release Pesticide Symp., 258, Wright State University, Dayton, OH (September 8-10, 1975).
13. Quisumbing, A.R., Lawatsch, D.J. and Kydonieus, A.F., Proc. Controlled Release Pesticide Symp., 247, Wright State University, Dayton, OH (September 8-10, 1975).
14. Sjogren, R.D., Proc. Controlled Release Pesticide Symp. 217, Wright State University, Dayton, OH (September 8-10, 1975).
15. Barnes, W.W. and Whitlaw, J.T., Preliminary Evaluation of Controlled Release Herbicide Formulations for Aquatic Weeds, Rep. U.S. Army Environ. Hygiene Agency, Edgewood, MD (Proj. 31-004-69/70) (1970).
16. Young, W.W. and Nelson, L.L., Evaluation of Controlled Release Herbicide Formulations for Aquatic Weeds, Entomol. Spec. Study No. 31-004-69/71, U.S. Army Environment Hygiene Edgewood, MD (July 1969 - July 1970).
17. Harris, F.W., Norris, S.O. and Post, L.K., Investigation of Factors Influencing Release of Herbicides from Polymer Matrices: The Polyethylene Matrix, Quart. Rep. II, Contract No. DACW 73-71-C-0053, U.S. Army Corps Engineers, (Oct. 1971-Dec. 1971).
18. Steward, K.K., Weed Investigations - Aquatic and Noncrop Areas Annual Rep., Agricultural Research Service, Ft. Lauderdale Fla., (July 1970 - June 1971).
19. Harris, F.W., Norris, S.O. and Post, L.K., Weed Sci., (1973) 21 (4), 318.
20. Harris, F.W., Feld, W.A. and Post, L.K., Investigation of Factors Influencing Release of Herbicides from Polymers Containing Herbicides as Pendent Side Chains. Annual Rep. Contract No. DACW 73-74-C-0001, U.S. Army Office Chief Engineer, Washington, D.C., (July 1973-June 1974).
21. Harris, F.W. and Post, L.K., Rep. No. 17, Proc. Controlled Release Pesticide Symp., University of Akron, Akron, OH, (September 16-18, 1974).
22. Bille, S., Mansdorf, S.F. and Cardarelli, N.F., Development of Slow Release Herbicide Materials for Controlling Aquatic Plants, Annual Rep. II to Dept. Army Office Chief Engineer, Contract No. DACW 73-70-C0030, (Nov. 1969 - July 1971) University of Akron, Product Development Lab., (July 1971).
23. Mansdorf, S.F., Rep. No. 12, Proc. Controlled Release Pesticide Symp., University of Akron, Akron, OH (September 16-18, 1974).
24. Abrams, J. and Hinkes, T.M., Pest Control, (May 1974) 14.
25. Jackson, W.M., Rep. No. 6, Controlled Release Pesticide Symp., University of Akron, Akron, OH (September 16-18, 1974).
26. Cornwall, P.B., International Pest Control (1970) 12 (4), 35.

27. Cardarelli, N.F. and Feldmesser, J., Proc. Controlled Release Pesticide Symp., 386, Wright State University, Dayton, OH (September 8-10, 1975).

27A. Feldmesser, J. Progress Report on Controlled Release of a Nematicide. Rep. No. 32, Proc. Controlled Release Pest. Symp. Akron, OH (Sept. 16-18, 1974).

28. Cardarelli, N.F., Evaluation of Incracide E-51 Against Select Aquatic Weeds and Algae, Rep. Creative Biology Lab., Proj. 104 to International Copper Research Assoc., New York, N.Y. (April 5, 1975).

29. Cardarelli, N.F. and Bille, S.M., Evaluation of Environmental Chemicals, Inc. Controlled Release Copper Sulfate, Rep. 1, Proj. 121, Creative Biology Lab., Barberton, OH, (March 1, 1976).

30. Hesketh, B., McKechnie Chemicals Ltd., Widnes, U.K., correspondence to Cardarelli, N., University of Akron, Akron, OH (13 February 1976).

31. Anon., Envirocap C., Chem. Eng. News (1972) 50 (23), 68.

32. Cardarelli, N.F., Dermal Protective Films, U.S. Patent 3,749,772 (1973).

33. Ivy, E.E., J. Econ. Entomol., (1972) 65, 473.

34. Selkirk, J., Envir. Action Bulletin, 3 (Oct. 2, 1976).

35. Hep, W.M. and Morrell, S.H., J. Appl. Chem., (1968) 18 (7), 189.

36. MacLachlin, J., Heap, W.M. and Pacitti, J., Monograph, Soc. Chemistry Industry, (1966) 23, 185.

37. Cardarelli, N.F., Weeds, Trees & Turf, (1972) 11 (5), 16

38. Janes, G.A., Bille, S.M. and Cardarelli, N.F., Development and Evaluation of Controlled Release Herbicides, Quart. Rep. U.S. Army Corps Engineers Contract No. DACW 39-76-C-0029 (Oct. 1 - Dec. 31, 1975).

5

Clinical Toxicology Aspects of Controlled Release Pesticide Formulations

JOHN DOULL

University of Kansas Medical Center, Kansas City, Kans. 66103

We are scheduled at this point in the program to consider some of the clinical toxicologic aspects of the controlled-release or microencapsulated pesticides. At the present time, however, there are no reported human cases of poisoning with microencapsulated pesticides, to my knowledge, and there is relatively little acute and chronic toxicity data available for these agents in animals. It is evident, therefore, that all we can do at this point in time is to speculate on how the use of these agents might affect the incidence and severity of pesticide poisoning in this country and to try to identify some of the problems that the emergency room physician may have to deal with in the event that these agents receive widespread commercial usage.

In looking back over the last 40 years at the incidence and causes of pesticide poisoning in this country, it seems to me that we have witnessed three more or less distinct phases in the epidemiology of pesticide poisoning and that we are now entering into what may be a fourth phase of this problem.

Pre-DDT Phase of Pesticide Poisoning

The first phase, which I designate as the pre-DDT era, was characterized by the heavy metals as the chief cause of pesticide poisoning with arsenic as the number one offender. Almost all of the agents which were used as pesticides during this period were highly toxic and this was true for the botanicals, such as strychnine and nicotine, as well as for the heavy metals, such as arsenic and lead. Although the use of these agents was moderate by today's standards, the toxicity of these agents made pesticide poisoning a significant problem in poison control. Even in those days, however, it was a relatively minor problem when compared with other agents that were responsible for poisoning cases. It has been estimated (1) that pesticides were responsible for between 5 and 10% of the cases of human poisoning during this pre-DDT phase and that the death rate was about 1 per million population.

DDT Phase of Pesticide Poisoning

The second phase of pesticide poisoning epidemiology began with the introduction of DDT in the 1940's and the subsequent addition of other chlorinated hydrocarbon insecticides in the 1950's. During this period there was a great increase in the use of pesticides in this country, but there was no corresponding increase in the number of human cases of pesticide poisoning (2). In fact, there were decreasing trends in both the absolute mortality and in the per cent incidence of poisoning during many portions of what I refer to as the DDT phase of pesticide poisoning epidemiology. Although the poison control statistics for this period were encouraging, they were not unexpected since we had anticipated that the replacement of highly toxic pesticides like arsenic and strychnine with agents like DDT, which is comparatively non-toxic following acute ingestion, would decrease the emergency room problem from pesticide poisoning. It was further anticipated that the mortality and morbidity associated with the older agents would decrease as they were replaced, and this also turned out to be true for both arsenic and strychnine (2). These trends were somewhat counteracted, however, by the growing problem of human poisoning with the organic phosphate insecticides and to a much lesser extent with the carbamate insecticides. It was apparent during the early 1960's, for example, that the organic phosphate insecticides were causing more occupational pesticide fatalities than any other class of agricultural chemicals and that in heavy use areas, like Florida and California, the organic phosphate insecticides were responsible for over half of the suicide deaths. In one year, for example, they caused more deaths in Dade County, Florida, than aspirin, which is traditionally our number one cause of poisoning in all areas (1).

Post-DDT Phase of Pesticide Poisoning

With the banning of DDT in the late sixties and the subsequent removal of other chlorinated hydrocarbon insecticides in the early seventies, we have entered into what I call the post-DDT or third phase of pesticide epidemiology. It is now almost 10 years since the appearance of the Mrak report in which the DDT ban was recommended. One of the things which was of real concern to several of us who participated in the preparation of this report was the likelihood that by eliminating DDT, farmers and other users would be forced to turn to substitutes which were far more toxic acutely and that, in effect, from the poison control viewpoint, we might have a situation where the cure was worse than the disease. Most emergency room physicians feel that this is exactly what has occurred (3).

Pesticides are very much like antibiotics in that the best agent or drug of choice is usually the one which exhibits a highly selective toxicity to the invading parasite or pest, yet is relatively non-toxic to the host or non-target species. When the physician is denied the use of a first-line antibiotic such as penicillin because of allergy or some other reason and forced to turn to a second-line drug such as vancomycin or even erythromycin, he expects to encounter more toxicity problems. Similarly, in replacing first-line pesticides like DDT or 2,4-D, which cause few acute toxicity problems with agents like parathion or paraquat, which present major treatment problems to the emergency room physician, it is unrealistic to expect that we can escape the consequences either in terms of the incidence of poisoning or in the severity of the cases which we see in the emergency room. The most recent data that we have obtained from the National Clearing House for Poison Control Centers suggests that insecticides are responsible for about half of all cases of pesticide poisoning, but there is no breakdown of this data into type of insecticide. In our own emergency room, insecticides accounted for about 71% of the pesticide contacts, but almost all of the pesticide poisoning cases which we treated were organic phosphate intoxications. We have had only one case of chlorinated hydrocarbon insecticide poisoning which required treatment in the past several months, and that was a 2-year-old girl who ingested Lindane.

Eldon Savage and his associates at the University of Iowa, the Medical University of South Carolina, and Colorado State University have recently published the results of their survey of hospitalized acute pesticide poisoning in the United States during the years of 1971, 1972, and 1973 (4). In this study, investigative teams were sent out to hospitals in both high and low pesticide use areas to collect demographic and hospital record information on both occupational and non-occupational cases of pesticide poisoning. Organophosphate insecticides were the leading cause of hospitalized pesticide poisoning in each of the three years surveyed for the occupational exposure group, but in the non-occupationally exposed group, which was mostly children under 5, the organophosphate insecticides were responsible for less than 20% of the poisoning cases. In interpreting this type of data, it should be kept in mind that patients who are hospitalized for symptoms of pesticide poisoning are more than twice as likely to die as those hospitalized for symptoms of other types of poisoning, and the difference is even more striking when one compares the outcome of different classes of pesticides or even different types of insecticides.

Prevention of Pesticide Poisoning

To return to the question of how microencapsulation may

affect pesticide poisoning in the future, we need to consider some of the current approaches to the problem of preventing pesticide poisoning. One approach would be to develop new pesticides which exhibit a much greater selective toxicity than the currently available pesticides. This principle has been used in developing antibiotics such as penicillin which kill the parasite by a mechanism which does not exist in the host or non-target organism and thereby provides a therapeutic index or safety margin of over 1000. Insect growth regulators and juvenile hormones are examples of agents in which an attempt is made to utilize a unique biological property of the insect to produce lethality and for which there may be no strict mammalian equivalent. Most previous attempts to develop this kind of absolute selective toxicity in pesticides have not been productive, but at least one of these juvenile hormones, methoprene, appears to be remarkably safe and environmentally harmless (5). Another related approach is to use insect sex pheromones and kairmones with a trapping system to reduce insect populations. Since it takes only a few molecules of these agents to produce their effect, it does not appear likely that their use will create serious acute poisoning problems. It has also been proposed to use chemosterilants, such as the alkylating agents, organotin and formamidines, for insect control, but since some of these agents produce serious toxic effects, there are at least potential poison control problems associated with their use. There is also a great deal of current interest in the use of integrated pest management practices as a possible solution to the pesticide poisoning problem and in the development of naturally occurring insecticides and new derivatives of older classes of insecticides, such as the pyrethroids (5). Although some of these approaches could have a significant impact on the problem of pesticide poisoning as seen in the emergency room, it looks like it is going to be quite some time before these approaches produce any significant change in either the incidence or type of poisoning that we are experiencing today.

There are, however, some other approaches which could have a more immediate impact. One of these which has been used abroad is to restrict the use of highly toxic pesticides such as parathion and methyl parathion, which cause more cases of organic phosphate insecticide poisoning than all of the rest of the agents in this class. This could be accomplished by simply banning selected agents as was done in Japan or by restricting the use of such agents to licensed pest control operators as proposed by the EPA. Eliminating all of the highly toxic agents, however, will not eliminate the problem of pesticide poisoning since poisoning can also occur with the less toxic agents provided the exposure is sufficiently great. As stated by Paracelsus, the father of toxicology, "All substances are poisons, thus dosage alone determines poisoning" (1). As a first step, however, we can solve the problem of pesticide poisoning in the user by insuring that all pesticides are formulated in such a way that it becomes impossible or virtually impossible for the user to be exposed to a toxic dose. We are already doing this to some extent in the drug area by the use of safety closures and limiting the quantity of agent in each container, and it has made a difference in the case of aspirin poisoning. We are already moving in this direction in the pesticide area by using granular formulations, low volume spray techniques, and synergizers which reduce the amount of pesticide needed in the formulation. It seems to me that microencapsulation of pesticides offers an interesting and potential method for achieving the same goal.

As an emergency room physician, I am appalled when I walk into my local hardware store and find that I can purchase bottles of pesticides formulated so that a single mouthful constitutes a lethal dose. I am not particularly reassured by the fact that each of these bottles contains a warning label describing the hazards associated with exposure to the pesticide, since most of our poisoning cases occur in children under five who can't read, or are intended suicides who use the label warning as a basis for their suicide attempt. Changes in our formulation practices may not prevent pesticide poisoning in the workers engaged in the manufacture and formulation of pesticides, and it may not be practical as a solution to the problem of occupational pesticide poisoning in agriculture, but it would certainly reduce the problem in our emergency room and that of other urban medical centers.

Possible Toxicologic Problems with Microencapsulated Pesticides

If we look at our previous experience with granular formulations of pesticides, it would appear that the microencapsulated pesticides should be more effective in reducing the incidence of pesticide poisoning following dermal and inhalation exposure than with ingestion. However, in patients who ingest granular formulations of pesticides, the symptoms generally develop more slowly and are less severe than those seen in patients who ingest pesticide concentrates. Gastric lavage and antidotal treatment are usually more efficacious in such cases in reducing the amount of pesticide absorbed and in preventing the subsequent symptoms. Removal of the granular material by lavage or emesis sometimes presents problems because of the tendency of the granules to form concretions in the stomach. It is also possible that the use of the microencapsulated pesticide formulation in an enclosed area could, over a long period of time, produce an inhalation hazard to occupants of the area. I would also be concerned about the possibility of an individual ingesting the microencapsulated pesticide together with a solvent or emulsifier which might facilitate the release of the pesticide. Although the microencapsulation process would not be expected to interfere with the antidotal efficacy of the currently available pesticide antidotes or with the usual therapeutic regimes used in the management of poisoning, this possibility should be investigated prior to their commercial use.

In a very real sense, the emergency room physician is at the end of a long developmental process, and by the time he has to deal with the problem, the toxicology is a closed book, the tolerances have been set, and the chemists are all off looking for a new agent. It seems to me that we need a more enlightened approach to the development of new pest control measures which would recognize that both accidental and intentional exposure to the agent will occur and includes, therefore, a specific effort along the way to figuring out how such patients should be handled. It is a lot easier to treat a poisoning when the management is preplanned and tested than when it is dictated by a crisis situation involving an unknown agent. I thank you for inviting me to participate at this early stage.

Literature Cited

1. Murphy, S. D., "Pesticides" In: Toxicology, the Basic Science of Poisons, Eds. L. J. Casarett and J. Doull, Macmillan Publishing Co., New York, N. Y., 1975.
2. Hayes, W. J., "Recognized and Possible Effects of Pesticides in Man" In: Toxicology of Pesticides, Ed. W. J. Hayes, Williams and Wilkins, Baltimore, Md., 1975.
3. Doull, J., "The Treatment of Insecticide Poisoning" In: Insecticide Biochemistry and Physiology, Ed. C. F. Wilkinson, Plenum Publishing Co., New York, N. Y., 1976.
4. Savage, E. P., "A Study of Hospitalized Acute Pesticide Poisoning in the United States", 1971 to 1973" EPA Contract 68-02-1271 and 68-01-3138, 1975.
5. Woods, J. S., Ed., Conference on Human Health Effects of New Approaches to Insect Pest Control, Environmental Health Perspectives (1976) 14: 1-193.

6

Matrix Factors Affecting the Controlled Release of Pesticides from Elastomers

N. F. CARDARELLI and S. V. KANAKKANATT

Environmental Management Laboratory, University of Akron, Akron, Ohio 44325

It is well known that various organic materials utilized as pest control agents are soluble in elastomers. If the solution limit is not exceeded, solute molecules are uniformly dispersed throughout the matrix in accordance with the principles governing solution equilibrium. During environmental exposure agent molecules adsorbed on the elastomer surface or absorbed just below that surface will pass via dissolution processes into the surrounding air, soil, or water. This action effectively creates a condition of localized disequilibrium and solute molecules, driven by solution pressure, migrate towards the depleting surface. Thus a continuous loss process is established. The mechanism has been treated at length by various authors[1-4]. Biologically efficacious longevity of such systems has been known to exceed nine years.[2] Present commercial applications are in the areas of antifouling coatings and long lasting molluscicides.[5-7]

In general, work with controlled release materials has been keyed to practical applications and based upon an empirical approach. The diffusion-dissolution mechanism has been elucidated but very little past effort has been devoted to the development of a fundamental understanding regarding the influence of compounding variables and matrix selection on the loss mechanism. Such knowledge would be of considerable value to the design of controlled release pesticide formulations and the optimization of favorable or desirable properties. The work reported herein is a step in that direction.

General Considerations

Proper compounding of the controlled release formulation is essential to develop various desirable properties - long half-life, appropriate agent loss rate, integrity of the processed geometry and the like. Experience has shown that the nature of the matrix, degree of crosslinking and the use of additives such as curatives, accelerators, reinforcing agents, antioxidants, etc. greatly influence agent solubility and loss rate. The cure system used affects both the rate of crosslinking and the ultimate crosslink density.

Carbon black and possibly other reinforcing additives tend to decrease the surface loss rate of the pesticide by increasing the diffusion path length. It may appear that the particle size of carbon black utilized is as critical as the amount. But fine blacks do not retard or prevent diffusion to any greater degree than coarse carbon blacks within the limits studied. In general, increasing the overall molecular weight and/or decreasing the molecular weight between crosslinks will lower the diffusion coefficient thus slowing loss rate.[8]

The segmental motion of a polymer chain increases as the temperature rises or when the ambient temperature is very far removed from the glass-transition temperatures (Tg) and the test temperature would be much above it. Variation in the environmental temperatures (T) alters the magnitude of the difference, T - Tg.

Two distinct volume fractions must be considered in a thorough study. One consists of the volume fraction of the rubber in the swollen state, arising from pesticide incorporation. This volume fraction reflects the original concentration of the pesticide. The other fraction consists of that volume of rubber containing the carbon black additive.

The variation of the above parameters is not entirely linear. However, for simplicity and the narrow limits of variation envisioned, the assumption of linearity appears to be justifiable. Serious departures from linearity are covered in this treatment by approximate correction factors.

Properties such as crystallinity, diffusant geometry, molecular weight of the starting elastomer, and interactions between additives are not considered at this time. Thus it is necessary to have a reference formulation. Based upon diffusion data obtained with the reference material, new formulations can be designed to provide a predicted release rate.

Theoretical Treatment

The following equations, used herein, have been previously derived:[8]

(1) $D_f = (2/3-V_r)\{D_o + \gamma[(T_2-T_{g_2}) - (T_1-T_{g_1})] - [\alpha - \delta(V_{s_2}-V_{s_1})]\ (d_{c_2}-d_{c_1})\}$

(2) $D_f = D_o + \gamma[(T_2-T_{g_2}) - (T_1-T_{g_1})] - [\alpha + \delta(V_{s_2}-V_s)]\ (dc_2-dc_1) - \beta(bc_2-bc_1)$

where: D_f = final diffusion coefficient. Subscripts 1 and 2 represent the equation number.
D_o = original diffusion coefficient
V_r = volume fraction of rubber in the carbon black filled formulation.
V_{s_1}, V_{s_2} = two different volume fractions of the pesticide - polymer composite.
T_1, T_2 = two different environmental temperatures.
T_{g_1}, T_{g_2} = glass transition temperatures of the two polymers.
α = cross-linking density coefficient.
β = carbon black content coefficient.
γ = temperature coefficient.
δ = slope of the curve α versus V_s.

Experimental Models

In order to validate the theoretical equations three groups of materials were examined. Three standard controlled release molluscicides in a chloroprene matrix are shown in table I, along with a control; series AA compounds consisting only of an elastomer and a peroxide curative; and series EB natural rubber compounds wherein the type and quality of carbon black were studied.

TABLE I
STANDARD MOLLUSCICIDE FORMULATIONS
(Cured at 300°F for 60 minutes)

Ingredient	Recipe (by parts per hundred parts elastomer) PDL-1	CBL-4	CBL-49A	CBL-3A
Chloroprene[1]	100	100	100	100
Zinc Oxide	5	5	5	5
Magnesium oxide	4	4	4	4
FEF Black[2]	14	14	14	---
HAF Black[3]	---	---	---	15
PBNA[4]	1	1	1	1
MBT[5]	---	1	---	---
Lauric Acid	3	3	3	3
TBTO[6]	---	8	---	---
TBTF[7]	---	---	---	8
DS649[8]	---	---	10	---

TABLE II
SERIES AA COMPOUNDS
(Cured at 300°F for 50 minutes)

Ingredient	Recipe (by parts per hundred parts rubber) AA-001	AA-002	AA-003
Polybutadiene[9]	100	---	---
Natural Rubber	---	100	---
Butyl Rubber[10]	---	---	100
Styrene-butadiene Copolymer[11]	---	---	---
Chloroprene[12]	---	---	---
Nitrile Rubber[13]	---	---	---
	AA-004	**AA-005**	**AA-006**
Polybutadiene[9]	---	---	---
Natural Rubber	---	---	---
Butyl Rubber[10]	---	---	---
Styrene-butadiene Copolymer[11]	100	---	---
Chloroprene[12]	---	100	---
Nitrile Rubber[13]	---	---	100

TABLE III
SERIES EB COMPOUNDS
(Cured at 300°F for 5 minutes)

Ingredient	Recipe (by parts per hundred parts rubber) CB-001	EB-001	EB-002
Natural Rubber	100	100	100
DICUP[14]	1.6	1.6	1.6
HCCB[15]	---	---	---
FEF	---	4	8
MT[16]	---	---	---

	EB-003	EB-004	EB-005
Natural Rubber	100	100	100
DICUP[14]	1.6	1.6	1.6
HCCB[15]	---	14	---
FEF	14	---	---
MT[16]	---	---	14

Notes

1. Neoprene WRT
2. Carbon black, 79 mμ average particle size
3. Carbon black 40 to 45 mμ average particle size
4. Phenyl-B-naphthylamine
5. Mercaptobenzothiazole
6. bis(tri-n-butyltin) oxide
7. Tributyltin fluoride
8. 3,3,4,4, tetrachlorotetrahydrothiophene pyridine 1,1-dioxide
9. Polybutadiene
10. Butyl rubber
11. Styrene-butadiene copolymer (SBR Plioflex)
12. Neoprene WRT
13. Nitrile rubber
14. Dicumyl peroxide
15. Carbon black, 15 mμ average particle size
16. Carbon black, 256 mμ average particle size

Release Rate Study

Specimens of the standard molluscicide compounds were cut from cured sheets at 2.5 x 2.5 x 0.15 cm, washed in distilled water and suspended in 400 ml of water. Samples were mechanically shaken at a constant rate throughout the experiment. Immersion water was evaporated to concentrate the agent and the amount of pesticide released determined analytically.

Diffusion Coefficient Determination

The diffusion coefficients for the AA and EB Series were determined by both sorption and desorption techniques. In the former method the sample is immersed in the sorpting liquid and weight gain noted at regular time intervals. The latter technique consisted of preswelling the specimen to equilibrium, removing from the liquid medium and periodically noting weight loss as a continuous air stream was passed over the surface. In a correlary study swollen test specimens were exposed at varying temperatures in a low vacuum oven and weight loss determined.

Results and Discussion

It is apparent from the results shown in Table IV that the presence of extremely hydrophobic agents (TBTO and TBTF) reduce water absorption whereas CBL-49A containing a hydrophillic agent (DS649) resulted in an increased water absorption rate.

TABLE IV[9]
DIFFUSION COEFFICIENT DETERMINATION
BY WATER ABSORPTION

Material	Molluscicide	Type	Diffusion Coefficient cm^2/sec
CBL-49A	DS-649	hydrophillic	2.1×10^{-8}
PDL-1	None	------------	5.0×10^{-9}
CBL-4	TBTO	hydrophobic	9.4×10^{-10}
CBL-3A	TBTF	hydrophobic	4.0×10^{-10}

In the study of the effect of the glass transition temperature (Tg) on the diffusion coefficient, (see Table V), n-decane was used as the desorbing liquid. The decrease in diffusion coefficient with increasing Tg is consistent with the known theories of diffusion. The dependence of D on Tg can be generally represented by use of the difference between T (test temperature) and Tg. Thus the effect of environmental temperature variation is incorporated in the governing equations by use of the T-Tg parameter.

TABLE V
EFFECT OF GLASS TRANSITION TEMPERATURE ON DIFFUSION COEFFICIENT

Material	Matrix	Tg(°C)	Diffusion Coefficient cm^2/sec
AA-001	Polybutadiene	-109	6.6×10^{-7}
AA-002	Natural Rubber	-70	2.99×10^{-7}
AA-003	Butyl Rubber	-65	1.3×10^{-7}
AA-004	Styrene-butadiene	-61	1.27×10^{-7}
AA-005	Chloroprene	-49	0.5×10^{-7}
AA-006	Nitrile	-24	0.1×10^{-7}

The effects of test temperature and carbon black content are depicted in Table VI. Two trends are apparent: (1) Diffusion coefficient increases with rising temperature, and (2) increasing carbon black content decreases D. Carbon black particle size is seemingly unimportant to n-decane diffusion.

TABLE VI[9]
EFFECT OF TEST TEMPERATURE AND CARBON BLACK CONTENT ON DIFFUSION COEFFICIENT IN NATURAL RUBBER

Material	Carbon Black Content (pphr)	Particle Size, nm	Diffusion Coefficient (10^{-6} cm^2/sec)			
			26°C	46°C	70°C	90°C
CB-001	0	--	3.08	4.02	5.42	7.00
EB-001	4	79	2.20	3.10	4.35	5.90
EB-002	8	79	1.91	2.70	3.80	4.96
EB-003	14	79	1.82	2.31	3.11	3.98
EB-004	14	15	1.86	2.25	2.99	3.66
EB-005	14	256	1.70	2.10	2.81	3.33

The molecular weights of the chain segments between crosslinks, M_c, have been determined by the equilibrium swelling method. Figure 1 depicts the dependence of the diffusion coefficient on temperature and M_c. D is plotted against T-Tg for matrices of varying M_c. The diffusion coefficient increases as T-Tg and Mc increase.

Computer Analysis

A computer assisted analysis of equations (1) and

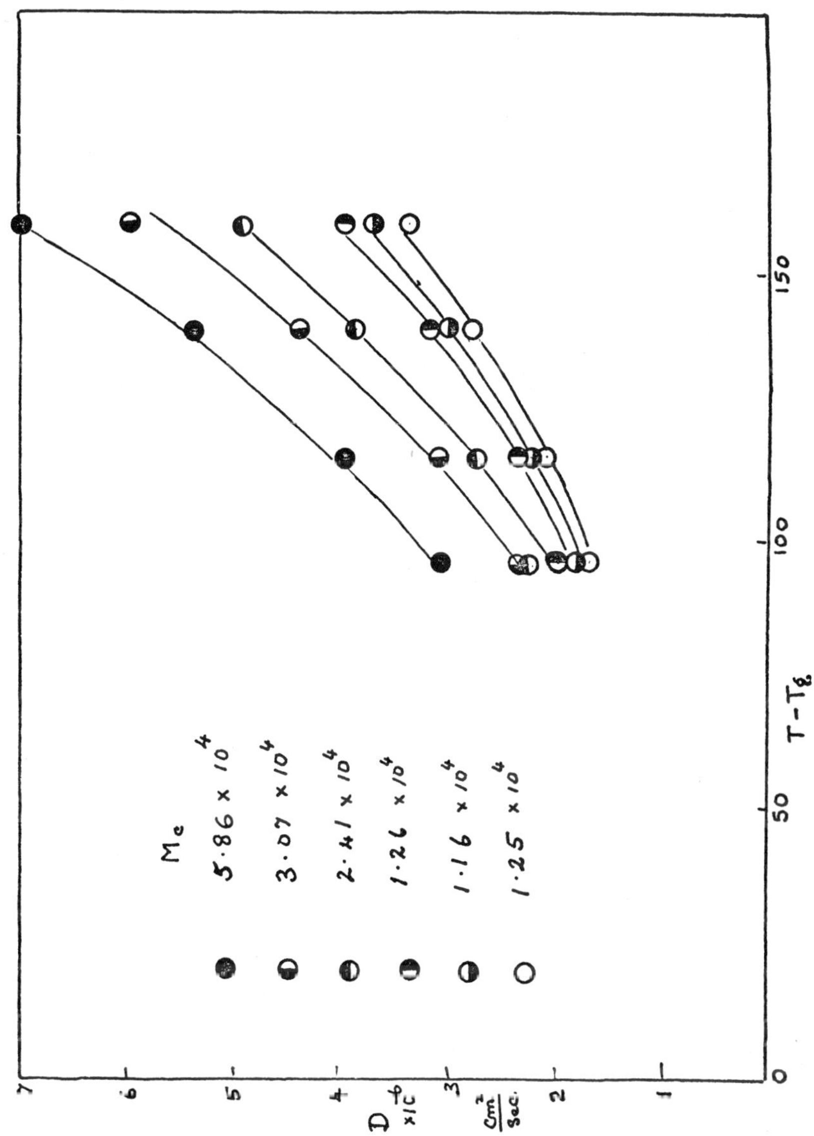

Figure 1. Curves showing the variation of the diffusion coefficient with M_c and T − T_g

(2) was undertaken. Complete treatment of all 13 variables was not possible; so several were held constant. They were:

$$D_o = C_1$$

$$\gamma = C_2$$

$$\alpha = C_3$$

$$\delta = C_4$$

$$\beta = C_5$$

The following single, or groups of variables were handled as shown:

$$V_r = X_1$$

$$(T_2 - Tg_2) - (T_1 - Tg_1) = X_2$$

$$Vs_2 - Vs_1 = X_3$$

$$dc_2 - dc_1 = X_4$$

$$bc_2 - bc_1 = X_5$$

Thus equations (1) and (2) reduce to (3) and (4) respectively:

(3) $Y_1 = 2/3 - X_1 \ (C_1 + C_2X_2) - (C_3 + C_4X_3) \ X_4$

(4) $Y_2 = C_1 + C_2X - (C_3 + C_4X_3) \ X_4 - C_5X_5$

where Y represents D_f

A complete program was composed to plot curves for equations (3) and (4) wherein X_1, X_2, X_3, X_4 and X_5 were varied one at a time.[10] A few of the hundreds of completed plots are presented.

The effects of diffusant concentration, temperature and carbon black content are illustrated in figures 2 and 3. In figure 2, it is evident that the diffusion coefficient, Y_1, increases as the diffusant concentration, reflected by X_3, increases. Also Y_1 rises as X_2, which reflects higher ambient temperature, a lower Tg, or both, increases. A similar trend is noted in figure 3. By comparing figures 2 and 3 it is evident that increasing the carbon black content reduces the diffusion coefficient; i.e., in figure 3

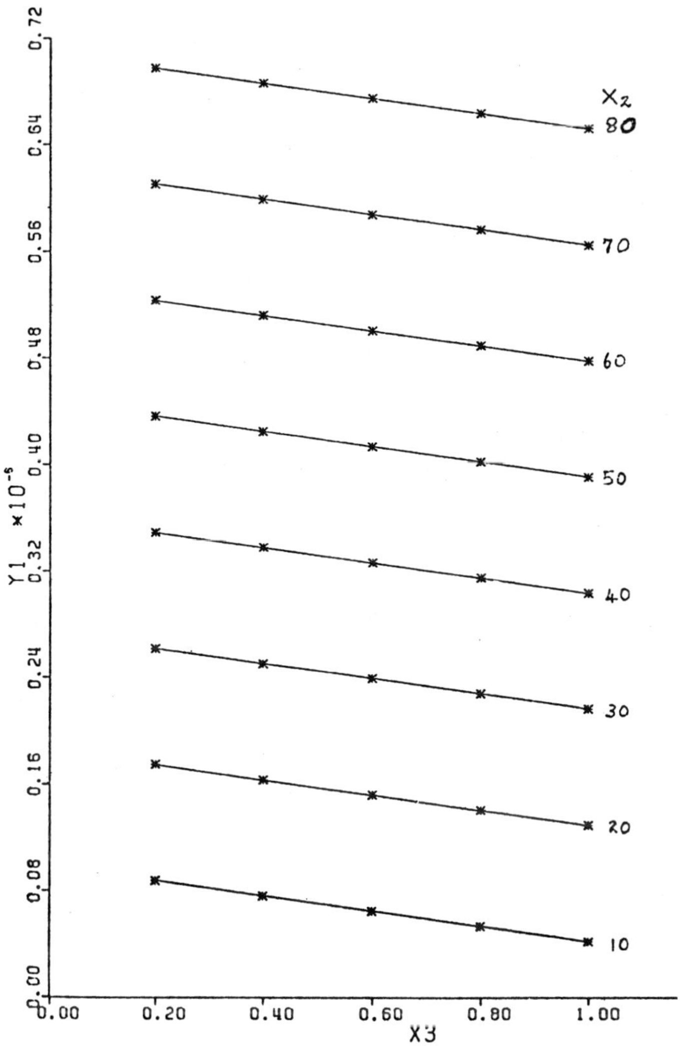

Figure 2. The plot of Y_1 vs. X_3 where $X_1 = 0.2$ and $X_4 = 1 \times 10^{-4}$

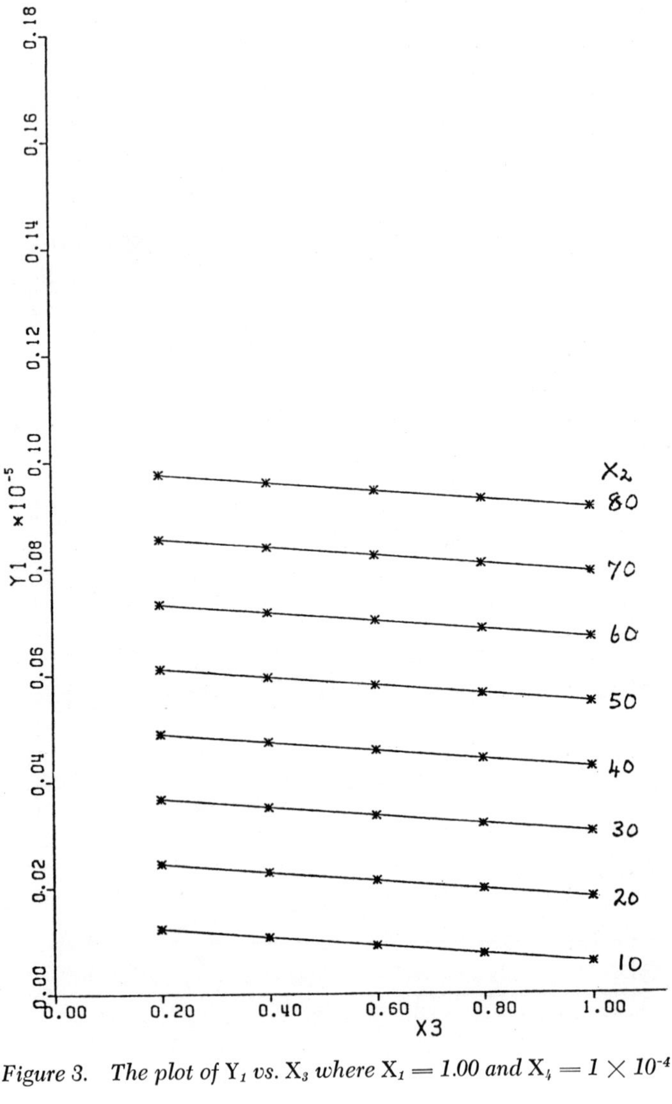

Figure 3. The plot of Y_1 *vs.* X_3 *where* $X_1 = 1.00$ *and* $X_4 = 1 \times 10^{-4}$

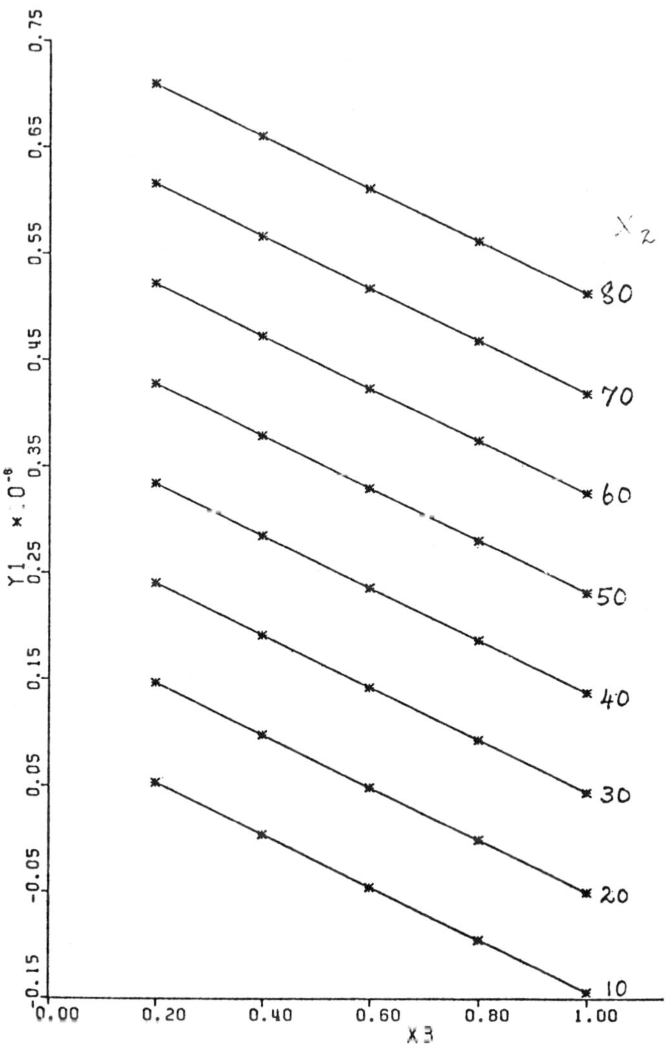

Figure 4. The plot of Y_1 vs. X_3 where $X_1 = 0.2$ and $X_4 = 4 \times 10^{-4}$

X_1 = 1 indicates no carbon black and in figure 2, X_1 = 0.2 means an 80% black content.

The effect of crosslink density is clearly seen by comparing figures 2 and 4. Note that the suppression of D is more pronounced at lower temperature and lower diffusant concentrations. At higher values of these variables, D is relatively unaffected--even with a fourfold increase in crosslink density.

Conclusions

Both experimental and computer methods of testing the validity of equations (1) and (2) indicate that they are adequate for prediction of the diffusion coefficient and release rate from a given formulation. Although several variables not incorporated in the derived equations have a definite effect on release rate, the equations and computer drawn curves can be used as guides to design formulations with the appropriate release rates for a particular application.

Abstract

Diffusion controlled release of the active agent is effectively used to deliver a pesticide from elastomeric matrices to the insect habitat. The rate of release is influenced by the nature of the elastomer as well as the conditions of the environment. Some of these influencing factors are considered and equations to estimate the diffusion coefficient are derived. A computer evaluation of these equations is attempted.

Literature Cited

1. Paul, D. R., and Harris, F. W., eds, Controlled Release Polymeric Formulations, ACS Symp. Ser. 33, ACS, Wash., D.C., 1976.
2. Cardarelli, N. F., "Controlled Release Pesticides Formulations," CRC Press, Cleveland, OH, 1976.
3. Higachi, I., Mechanisms of Sustained Action Medication, J. Pharm. Sci. 52, 1145, 1963.
4. Collins, R. L., A Theoretical Foundation For Slow Release, Proc. Controlled Release Pesticide Symp., Rep. 9, Univ. Akron, Akron, OH, Sept. 16-18, 1974.
5. Cardarelli, N. F. and Caprette, S. J., Antifouling Covering, U.S. Patent 3,426,473, 1969.
6. Cardarelli, N. F. and Neff, H. F., Biocidal Elastomeric Compositions, U.S. Patent 3,639,583,

1972.
7. Cardarelli, N. F., Biocidal Elastomeric Composition and Method for Dispersing Pesticides Therewith, U.S. Patent 3,851,053, 1974.
8. Kanakkanatt, S. V., The Effect of Matrix Properties on the Diffusion Coefficient of Liquids Through Rubber, Macromol. Reprint, 1, 614, 1971.
9. Kanakkanatt, S. V., Schistosomiasis Control By Slow Release Molluscicides, Product Development Lab., Univ. Akron, Report to World Health Organization (Unpub.), Sept. 15, 1972.
10. Kanakkanatt, S. V., Influence of Formulation Properties on the Diffusion-Dissolution Mechanism, Proc. Controlled Release Pesticide Symp. 8.42, Univ. Akron, Akron, OH, Sept. 13-15, 1976.

7

Encapsulation of Pesticides within a Starch Matrix

W. M. DOANE, B. S. SHASHA, and C. R. RUSSELL

Northern Regional Research Center, Agricultural Research Service, U.S. Department of Agriculture, Peoria, Ill. 61604

At the Northern Regional Research Center, a research program is directed towards developing agriculturally based raw materials as renewable resources for chemicals to replace in part those derived from petroleum. Starch, a polysaccharide produced in great abundance in nature, is a prime candidate as a raw material because of its availability and relatively low cost and because it can be converted readily into a variety of useful monomeric and polymeric products by chemical and biochemical means. A low-cost derivative, starch xanthate, is useful in papermaking applications (1), for reinforcement of rubber (2), in making powdered rubber (3), and for removing heavy metals from polluted water (4). Because of the ease with which starch xanthate can be insolubilized from an aqueous solution by crosslinking under mild oxidation conditions or with metal cations, and because of the film-forming nature of certain crosslinked products, we explored the possibility of using this material as an encapsulating matrix for pesticides. We envisioned that release of a lipophilic pesticidal chemical from a hydrophilic but water-insoluble starch matrix would be slow and could be controlled to a considerable degree by simple modifications. Such a matrix would have an added advantage of being biodegradable and thus would leave no residue in the environment.

A preliminary report (5) described our first attempts to utilize oxidatively coupled starch xanthate (xanthide) as a slow-release matrix for pesticides and suggested that such a system was worthy of further research in attempts to optimize release characteristics. We now wish to report the results of our further studies and data from preliminary field tests with selected formulations.

The procedure based on starch xanthate consists of dispersing the active agent in an aqueous starch xanthate solution and subsequently crosslinking the starch xanthate either oxidatively, or with multivalent metal ions, or with difunctional reagents such as epichlorohydrin. Cereal flours, which contain about 10% protein along with starch, also can be xanthated and used as an encapsulating matrix. Upon crosslinking, which is effected within a few seconds under ambient conditions, the entire mass becomes gellike and, on continued mixing for an additional few seconds, becomes a particulate solid which can be dried to low moisture content with only minimal or no loss of the entrapped chemical. That only a single phase is produced on crosslinking with no supernatant is important in assuring essentially complete entrapment of both water-soluble and water-insoluble pesticidal chemicals.

Other polymers can be incorporated readily into the products as a means to modify release properties. Polymers like polystyrene, polyethylene, and poly(vinyl chloride) are just dissolved in a small amount of an appropriate solvent such as benzene or acetone then added to the xanthate solution. Poly(styrene-butadiene), commercially provided as a latex, is conveniently added in this form. Upon crosslinking the xanthate, the other polymers are entrapped along with the active agents.

Another modification easily made which can modify release properties provides products which are doubly encapsulated. This is achieved on addition of more starch xanthate, either alone or containing another polymer, after the initial crosslinking reaction has been effected and then adding additional crosslinking agent.

The starch xanthate used for encapsulation is prepared under ambient conditions by treating a water suspension of starch with carbon disulfide and an alkali metal hydroxide. Typically about 70% of the carbon disulfide is converted to xanthate within 30 minutes with little or no additional conversion occurring on prolonged standing. Although the theoretical number of xanthate groups possible for each anhydroglucose repeating unit of starch is 3 [degree of substitution (DS) of 3], we find that a DS of 0.1 to 0.35 is sufficient. Viscosity of xanthate solutions increases proportionally with DS and starch xanthate concentration. When whole unmodified starch (regular pearl starch) is used as the starting material, a starch xanthate concentration of near 15% is about the maximum that can be handled for the encapsulation process. Higher concentrations, usable in this process, of up to nearly 60% can be achieved, if the starting starch is reduced in molecular size by hydrolysis of some of the glucopyranosyl linkages with acids or enzymes.

Such modifications are conventional commercial procedures designed to provide degraded starch products for a variety of industrial uses.

Use of the more concentrated starch xanthate solutions has an obvious advantage in cost for drying the particulate encapsulated product. However, there are certain limitations on using the highly concentrated solutions. The amount of active agent that can be effectively encapsulated within the crosslinked starch xanthate matrix is inversely proportional to starch xanthate concentration. For example, when starch xanthate of 14% concentration is used, a final product is obtained which contains a maximum of 47% of a liquid thiocarbamate. When 50% xanthate is employed the maximum is reduced to 13%.

The values conceivably might vary with the nature of the chemical to be encapsulated. For the examples given, the active agent was butylate* (S-ethyl diisobutylthiocarbamate). At the highest level, where the particulate product consists of nearly 50% of the highly volatile liquid butylate, the particles have a wetted appearance and are not completely free flowing. At about 40% or less, they appear dry and give a free-flowing product.

Although various methods have been employed for crosslinking the xanthate with apparently similar results, we have worked mostly with the oxidative method and have used either nitrous acid or hydrogen peroxide as the selected oxidant. Both oxidants effectively crosslink the xanthate to xanthide (starch-O-$\overset{\text{S}}{\overset{\|}{\text{C}}}$-S-S-$\overset{\text{S}}{\overset{\|}{\text{C}}}$-O-starch) at a pH of 4 to 5. Since the xanthate is made under alkaline conditions, the pH must be lowered to allow crosslinking. For pesticides, which are labile to alkali, the pH can be adjusted to near neutrality before addition of the active agent. For the nitrous acid system, sodium nitrite is added to the alkaline xanthate solution and becomes the active oxidant when the pH is lowered to 4-5. When peroxide is used, it is added to a neutralized xanthate and then pH is lowered further. Only slightly more than stoichiometric amounts of oxidant are required, and since the oxidation proceeds to completion rapidly, even active agents which are susceptible to oxidation are not likely to be oxidized during encapsulation. Although

---

* This paper reports the results of research only. Mention of a pesticide in this paper does not constitute a recommendation for use by the U.S. Department of Agriculture nor does it imply registration under FIFRA as amended. Also, mention of firm names does not constitute an endorsement by the U.S. Department of Agriculture over other firms not mentioned.

both oxidants appear to work equally well in crosslinking the xanthate, encapsulated products are quite different in appearance and in release properties of the active agent. Nitrous acid crosslinked products contain numerous microscopic openings in the matrix, due apparently to small amounts of nitrous oxide gas generated during the reaction. These openings result in a relatively rapid rate of release as will be described later. The peroxide-coupled products are without visible openings and provide much slower release of active agent.

Shelf life of the starch-encapsulated pesticides is good, and there is no appreciable loss on storage in closed containers during 1 year. When placed in open containers for several days, loss of volatile agent is negligible. However, when products are wetted or immersed in water, active agent is then released from the matrix. We devised a simple laboratory screening test for comparing release properties of thiocarbamate- containing products to assist in selection of formulations for subsequent bioassay. The test consists of placing several 1-gram portions of a product in watch glasses placed in a hood and applying to each 2-ml of water. The water slowly evaporates during a 24-hour period in the hood. Then water is again added and the wetted product again allowed to stand for 24 hours. This repeated wetting and drying is continued for the duration of the test with entire 1-gram samples being removed periodically and analyzed for total nitrogen content in those instances where the active agent contains nitrogen. Table I shows the release characteristics for four different formulations containing butylate.

Table I
Release Properties of Butylate Formulations

Xanthate base[a]	Loss of butylate, % 1 day	2 days	8 days
Acid-modified flour[b]	29	58	68
Acid-modified flour-starch mixture[c]	20	36	48
Starch[c]	0	0	8
Starch + 20% latex[c]	0	0	37
None (control)	68	98	100

[a] Xanthate DS was 0.35 and double encapsulation was used for each.
[b] $NaNO_2$ used for oxidation.
[c] H_2O_2 used for oxidation.

It would appear that either the protein component in the flour or the lower molecular weight of the starch component of the flour contributes to a faster release of butylate; however, this remains to be confirmed. Other preliminary tests indicate that DS of xanthate, e.g., crosslink density of the matrix, may play a significant role in controlling release of active agent, and studies to confirm this are underway.

Depending on the amount of shear placed on the particulate product before drying, a range of particle sizes can result. With simple hand mixing, a particle size of 14 mesh or larger is typically obtained. For small laboratory preparations, we shear the wet product in a Waring Blendor for a few seconds to produce smaller particle sizes.

We have not as yet attempted to provide products fine enough to pass 100 mesh. Grinding or milling the dried products can yield fine powders but considerable amounts of pesticide are lost, especially if they are highly volatile ones. Whereas shearing of the wet product results mostly in breaking up the agglomerates composed of several smaller particles, grinding or milling of dry products disrupts the matrix encapsulating the pesticide.

A product prepared from starch xanthate of DS 0.175 and crosslinked with H_2O_2 in the presence of EPTC (S-ethyl dipropylthiocarbamate) was dried and separated into four fractions by sieving. The four fractions were analyzed for active agent content and loss of agent after treatment with water for 2 days. Results are shown in Table II.

Table II
Properties of Starch Xanthide-EPTC Formulations as Related to Particle Size

Mesh size	% of Total	EPTC, %	Loss of EPTC after water treatment, % of total
>60	5	14.0	14
30-60	10	21.7	17
14-30	70	21.7	5
<14	15	21.7	5

Except for the 5% fraction which passed 60 mesh, there was no difference in the amount of pesticide contained in the particles of various sizes. It does appear that smaller size particles release EPTC at a faster rate.

Some of the formulations we have prepared have been evaluated by others in various laboratory bioassay tests and, in one instance, in replicated field plots. Although the data obtained are encouraging and indicate considerable promise for the starch technology, it should be understood that the data are preliminary and that the formulations tested are by no means the optimum formulations that can be developed. That the release properties of various pesticides from the crosslinked starch or flour xanthate matrix can be considerably improved through minor modifications in the encapsulation process is strongly supported by our continuing research.

Feldmesser et al. (6) reported on laboratory evaluations of starch xanthide formulations of DBCP (1,2-dibromo-3-chloropropane), a nematicide, and diazinon [O,O-diethyl O-(2-isopropyl-6-methyl-4-pyrimidinyl)] phosphorothioate, an insecticide-nematicide for nematicidal activity. Two DBCP formulations containing 35.6% and 42.0% active agent and two diazinon ones containing 42.0 and 43.6% active were studied. To determine retention of active agent under various conditions, the products were aerated both wet and dry in open dishes for several days and then amount retained was determined by bioassays against nematodes in a standard *in vitro* test. During 10 days aeration of wet DBCP formulations, most of the active agent was lost and their subsequent effectiveness for killing nematodes was minimal. Retention of diazinon was considerably greater, perhaps due to its much lower vapor pressure than DBCP. During the 10-day aeration tests and an additional 34 days of aeration in the dry, the two diazinon formulations lost only about 20-33% of their active ingredient. The mortality of *Panagrellus rediviuus*, a saprophagous nematode, after 48 hours exposure to 200 ppm diazinon in the form of the two starch xanthide formulations after various periods of aeration is shown in Table III.

Cooperative work is continuing between Feldmesser's and our Laboratories in attempts to develop formulations capable of effectively killing nematodes over an extended period.

Whereas many herbicides must be incorporated in the soil soon after application to the surface to prevent extensive losses due to volatilization or decomposition by sunlight, it is hoped that controlled release formulations may prolong the time before incorporation is needed, or ideally, to provide control without being incorporated. Four formulations containing butylate prepared by us were evaluated in the laboratory by Stauffer Chemical Company for the ability to delay time before incorporation. Butylate as an emulsifiable concentrate (EC) was applied as a control. Rates of active agent (ai) of 3 and 4 lb/A were applied. Formulations were placed on the surface of wet soil and incorporated immediately and after 24 hours. Results are shown in Tables IV and V.

Table III
Release Properties of Starch Xanthide-Diazinon Formulation

	Percent kill			
	42.0%		43.6%	
	10 days	44 days	10 days	44 days
Starch-diazinon				
Wet[a]	69.4	63.0	76.3	52.5
Dry	66.2	63.1	75.4	70.0
Unaerated[b]	74.6	76.0	78.1	74.3
Technical diazinon				
Wet[a]	81.0	0	82.8	0
Dry	76.6	0	77.4	0
Unaerated[b]	89.0	0	95.1	0

[a] Second aeration period of 34 days following 10 day wet and dry aeration and 48 hours exposure was dry for all granules.
[b] Granules not aerated for first 10 days. Aerated dry for 34 days.

Table IV
Percent Weed Control[a] by Delayed Incorporation of Butylate Formulations

Formulation	Rate	Incorporation 0 Hours	Incorporation 24-Hour delay
SX-butylate[b]	3 lb ai/A	80	75
SX-butylate[c]	3 lb ai/A	85	67
Butylate (EC)	3 lb ai/A	87	10

[a] Average control of barley, foxtail, watergrass, wild oat, crabgrass, annual ryegrass, and shattercane.
[b] Starch xanthate of DS 0.3; $NaNO_2$ was used for crosslinking; about 25% butylate.
[c] Same as b except containing 35% butylate.

Table V
Percent Weed Control by Delayed Incorporation of Butylate Formulations

Formulation	Rate	Incorporation 0 Hours	Incorporation 24-Hour delay
SX-butylate[a]	4 lb ai/A	77	68
SX-butylate[b]	4 lb ai/A	79	69
Butylate (EC)	4 lb ai/A	82	28

[a] Starch xanthate of DS 0.3; $NaNO_2$ used for crosslinking; 25.5% butylate.
[b] Same as a except larger particle size.

Although the results are preliminary, a benefit is seen for the encapsulated products in allowing a longer time on the soil surface before incorporation.

Schreiber (7), at Purdue University, recently reported results of greenhouse and field tests of two starch xanthide-EPTC products. The formulations were made from starch xanthates of DS 0.35, and sodium nitrite was used for crosslinking. One formulation contained 14% EPTC and the other was a double-encapsulated product containing 20% latex polymer and 22% EPTC. In the greenhouse, the double-encapsulated product was compared with EPTC applied as the emulsifiable concentrate. The materials were applied to soils at a rate of 3 lb/A and were incorporated into soils seeded with robust purple foxtail.

At 31 days after seeding, the plants were removed and weighed and the pots reseeded. This procedure was repeated at 52 and 87 days and the final harvest was at 120 days. Results are shown in Table VI.

Table VI
Weed Control by Starch Xanthide-EPTC Formulation

Treatment	Yield, g/pot			
	31 Days	52 Days	87 Days	120 Days
Untreated	1.6	2.0	2.8	2.2
EPTC (EC)	0	0.1	2.7	2.8
Starch xanthide-EPTC	0	0.01	0.4	3.9

At 31 and 52 days, both the EC and the starch xanthide formulations gave excellent control of foxtail. However, between 52 and 87 days, the EC completely lost its effectiveness while the starch product still gave good control. Between 87 and 120 days, the starch product lost its effectiveness. The greater weight of plant material in both treated pots over the control is due to the greater fertility level remaining in the soil of these pots.

In the field, the EC, single-encapsulated and double-encapsulated products were applied at active ingredient levels of 3 and 6 lb ai/A, incorporated, and overseeded with yellow, giant, and giant green foxtail. Natural populations of pigweed, lambsquarter, smartweed, jimson, and velvetleaf were the dominant broadleaf weeds. Forty-seven days after application, weed stand counts and weed weights by species were made on each plot. Results are shown in Table VII.

Table VII
Weed Control by Single and Double Encapsulated EPTC Formulations

Treatment[a]	Total weed	
	Count	Weight, g
Untreated	95.3	924.8
EC-EPTC	48.0	247.8
Starch-EPTC (single)	33.7	186.0
Starch-EPTC (double)	33.0	31.0

[a] Applied at a rate of EPTC of 3 lb/A.

When applied at the 6 lb ai/A level, excellent control of all vegetation was obtained 105 days after treatment with the double-encapsulated formulations.

Cooperative work between Schreiber's Laboratory and ours is continuing with plans made for extensive field testing during 1977.

Literature Cited

1. Hamerstrand, G. E., Carr, M. E., Hofreiter, B. T., and Russell, C. R. Staerke (1976) 28(7):240-243.
2. Buchanan, R. A., Seckinger, H. L., Kwolek, W. F., Doane, W. M., and Russell, C. R. J. Elast. Plast. (1976) 8(1):82-95.
3. Abbott, T. P., James, C., Doane, W. M., and Russell, C. R. J. Elast. Plast. (1975) 7(2):114-132.
4. Wing, R. E., Doane, W. M., and Russell, C. R. J. Appl. Polym. Sci. (1975) 19(3):847-854.
5. Shasha, B. S., Doane, W. M., and Russell, C. R. J. Polym. Sci., Polym. Lett. Ed. (1976) 14(7):417-420.
6. Feldmesser, Julius, Shasha, B. S., and Doane, W. M. Proceedings 1976 Controlled Release Pesticide Symposium, Akron, Ohio, September 13-15, 1976, pp. 6.18-6.29.
7. Schreiber, Marvin. Efficacy and Persistence of Starch Encapsulated EPTC. Presented at the Northcentral Weed Control Conference, Omaha, Nebraska, December 7-9, 1976.

8

Controlled Release of Pesticides from Kraft Lignin Carriers

H. T. DELLICOLLI

Polychemicals Department, Westvaco Corp., N. Charleston, S. C. 29406

Constituting part of the cell wall of most dry land plants, lignin is the world's second most abundant aromatic polymer. In fact, lignin which is exceeded only by cellulose in abundance, is the primary non-petroleum source of the aromatic nucleus in nature.

Native lignin, or lignin as it exists in the living tree for example, imparts structural rigidity to stems of the plant by acting as a bonding agent between cells. It also plays a role in decreasing the permeation of water across cell walls in the vascular system of the tree and imparts resistance to attack by certain microorganisms, presumably because of its phenolic nature.

This material is produced in nature from the glucosides of coniferyl and sinapyl alcohols.

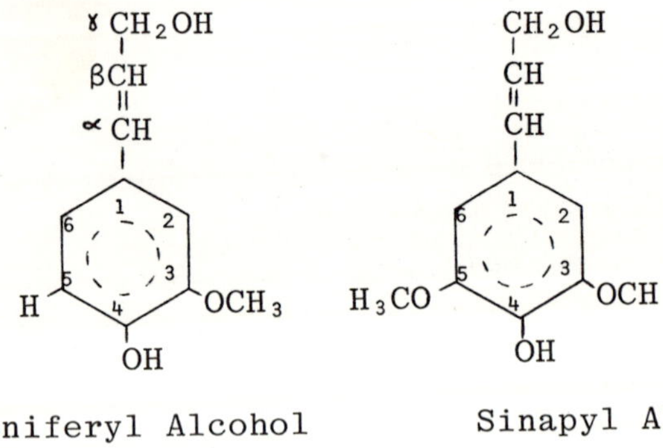

Coniferyl Alcohol Sinapyl Alcohol

The actual polymerization is proceeded by an enzymatic dehydrogeneration which leads to a free radical with electron density delocalized to the phenolic oxygen and carbons 5, 1, and β. According to Nimz (1) random coupling through each of these reactive sites leads to a natural material with a statistical distribution of at least ten different types of bonds.

Kraft Lignin

The form of kraft lignin to be discussed in the following pages however, is not the native lignin described above, but a product of the kraft pulping process. Here, the lignin in the wood is solubilized during the pulping process by particle depolymerization and incorporation of a solubilizing group to allow separation of lignin and hemicellulose from the cellulose fibers.

Technical kraft lignin is a polyphenolic material which is soluble in very alkaline aqueous solutions such as kraft pulping liquors, but highly insoluble in neutral or acidic media. This is in contrast to the lignosulfonates isolated as by-products of the sulfite pulping process which are soluble under neutral and moderately acidic conditions. Both sulfite lignins and sulfonated kraft lignins are used extensively in the agricultural chemical industry as anionic dispersants. They, just to name a few, have the familiar Marasperse, Maracarb, (American Can - sulfite), REAX and POLYFON (Westvaco-sulfonated kraft) tradenames.

The physical chemistry of kraft lignin is to say the least, a nebulous area, a situation due in part to the random and not yet fully understood mode of in vivo synthesis of the parent native lignin, the statistical distribution of its functionality and the changes in its structure and composition which take place during the pulping process.

Currently available data (2,3,4) indicate that aside from solubility in alkaline solutions as well as many polar organic solvents, technical kraft lignin has an intrinsic viscosity $\{\eta\}$= 6 ml/g. Other hydrodynamic data such as diffusion and sedimentation coefficients suggest a roughly spherical shape for the dissolved macromolecule. Number average molecular weights are 1600 and 1050 for pine and hardwood lignin respectively. This material is moderately polydisperse, $\bar{M}w/\bar{M}n$ = 2.2 for pine and 2.8 for hardwood (5).

Kraft Lignin as a Carrier for Controlled Release Pesticide

Kraft lignin appears to have several advantages over petrochemical based polymers as a potential carrier system for pesticides. The aromatic nature of lignin makes it an excellent protective matrix for biologically active materials sensitive to degradative processes initiated by ultraviolet radiation from sunlight. Secondly, the antioxidant properties of lignin would add further stability to the chemically unstable pesticides, a characteristic of many of the "non-persistant" agents in use today or being developed for future use. Lignin is biodegradable, a factor which in light of the current and undoubtedly future trends in chemical pest control makes this natural polymer highly desirable as a carrier. In the soil, lignin is microbially degraded by several microorganisms such as the white rot fungi belonging to the family Basidomycetes to precursors of humus, one of the few natural substances considered more ubiquitous than lignin itself. Several of the pathways of the degradation of lignin by microflora into humus were reviewed and described by Christman and Oglesby (6).

After all has been said and done about the performance of controlled release systems in the laboratory or in the greenhouse, the delivery system itself must be capable of being economically converted to a stable and usable formulation which can be utilized by its intended user, the farmer. If these forms or formulations are similar to the currently used systems such as emulsifiable concentrates, wettable powders, or granules, the controlled release formulation will appear less alien to the farmer and acceptance by the user will occur sooner than if the system required a major change in application practice. In light of the reeducation necessary for controlled release systems to gain general acceptance, any factor which will make this concept appear less alien will hasten the appearance of the time when the delivery system will find common use.

To this end, many lignin/pesticide systems have the capability of being converted to formulations such as those described above in the same equipment now used to produce conventional formulations of the these pesticides. For example, wettable powders have been prepared from simizine, pentachloronitrobenzene, hexachlorophene, methyl parathion controlled release composites and 2,4-D while granules incorporating several phenoxyacetics, substituted benzoic acids and carbamates have been produced in the laboratory. All of the above utilized carrier systems are based upon technical kraft lignin.

It became apparent, however, when several composites of technical kraft lignin and organophosphates such as Ethoprop (Mobil Chemical) and carbamates such as Bux (Chevron) took the form of viscous gums or deformable solids which could only be ground cyrogenically that the lignin was not universally acceptable as a carrier. Even after the low temperature grind, the formulations had absolutely no shelf stability. Both small particle formulations and granules either sintered within hours at temperatures as low as 30°C or in many cases actually liquified within days at slightly higher temperatures (< 50°C). These observations led to the development of a chemically modified lignin carrier prepared by modifying the parent technical kraft to produce a reversably swellable porous matrix. With few exceptions, this carrier made possible the preparation of stable formulations of those agricultural chemicals which plasticized the parent lignin.

In another instance, the lignin was converted to a second modification. The carrier system produced was again swellable, but underwent 11-fold volume increase upon hydration as compared to a two-fold change displayed by the previous carrier. This carrier was found useful for water soluble pesticides such as the amine salts of 2,4-D, etc.

The above modifications were made possible because of one of the major advantages of kraft lignin. This factor is its ability to be chemically modified. Work to be discussed in the ensuing paragraphs describe field results of these composites each of which employs one of the basic carriers described above. These experimental systems are kraft lignin/Terraclor (PCNB), modified lignin/Mocap (ethoprop), and modified lignin/2,4-D (dimethyl amine salt).

Carrier Selections.

While the choice of carrier systems for any given technical pesticide is still largely emperical, some insight into the extent which the carrier and active ingredient interact and plasticize kraft lignin can be gained by calculating the solubility parameter of the pesticide. Generally, estimation of this parameter with the structural group consideration of Small (7) will suffice. Experience has shown where δ for the pesticide falls between 10.5 and 12 $(cal/cm^3)^{1/2}$ the likelihood of plasticization is high. A value of δ=11.5 is used for technical kraft lignin.

Test results - Lignin - 2,4-D.

The first system tested consisted of a granular composite of chemically modified lignin with a loading of 10% by weight 2,4-D (as the dimethyl amine salt). Composites were prepared by placing the dry lignin based carrier is a solution of the 2,4-D salt, allowing it to swell and absorb all of the solution (500 grams of solution per 50 grams of lignin), drying and granulating the composite.

A series of soil filled trays divided into 1 $ft.^2$ compartments were placed on the windward side of a ditch bank immediately adjacent to a large weed covered field. It was intended that these trays catch windborne seed and allow it to germinate where no chemical was used or prevent germination where herbicide was employed. Controlled release composite was applied to ten trays as granules and conventional 2,4-D amine salt formulations as aqueous spray. Ten trays were left as controls (untreated). Herbicide was applied at the rate of ½ lb./acre for both controlled release and conventional formulations.

The test plots were examined monthly and all growing plants were removed. As a further check, 5 bean seeds were planted in each compartment and the total number of bean plants recorded at each evaluation, removed and then replanted.

Observations are recorded in the following table.

Table I
Field results of lignin/2,4-D (amine salt) controlled release granules

	Controlled Release		Conventional Formulation		Check	
Date	Weeds	Beans	Weeds	Beans	Weeds	Beans
April 1974	27	0	24	0	74	48
May 1974	20	0	31	0	96	45
June 1974	18	0	115	31	133	50
July 1974	27	0	241	50	237	50
August 1974	94	0	296	48	304	49
September 1974	86	26	251	50	276	49
October 1974	226	50	341	50	300	50

These data indicate that the controlled release form of 2,4-D did provide effective control of susceptable species for five months before losing activity while the conventional form of the same herbicide applied at the same rate lasted two months. A system such as this would find use perhaps as a preemergent broadleaf herbicide for winter grain crops.

Lignin - ethoprop.

A second field exercise involved the evaluation of lignin-ethoprop (Mocap) composites in the control of the root knot nematode. Because of its extreme sensitivity to both soil pests and phytotoxic chemicals, the cucumber was chosen as the test crop.

The composites were prepared using a modified lignin, PC-402, developed for use with organophosphates. Incorporation of the active material into the carrier was a matter of spraying the preheated carrier (80° C) with a solution of ethoprop in 95/5 (v/v) $\frac{\text{methylene chloride}}{\text{methanol}}$, evaporating the solvent and formulating as a microgranule (80-100 mesh). Carrier PC-402 was selected because earlier attempts to formulate with technical kraft lignin resulted in a system which could not be crushed because of its plastic consistency.

Field evaluation of the composites was carried out at the Clemson University Truck Experiment Station in Charleston, S. C. Initial data became available during the fall of 1974 and is presented in Table II.

Table II

Effect of nematocide formulations on the yield and on control of root-knot nematodes of cucumbers. (Fall 1974)

Treatment	Method of Application	Rate/Acre	Yield (bu/acre)	Root-Knot Index 1/
Control			210	3.0
Mocap	Broadcast	5.0 lbs.	180	2.8
Mocap-lignin composite	Broadcast	5.0 lbs.	210	1.6
Fumazone	Row	0.5 gal.	247	0.1

1/ Root-knot index = 0.0 (no root damage) - 5.0 (mass galls, decayed roots, etc.

This data indicates that the controlled release formulation applied at the same rate as the conventional formulation was more effective in controlling the target organism as indicated by a lower root-knot index. Only Fumazone was more effective than the controlled release system. An additional benefit derived from the controlled release formulation was a yield increase attributed to a reduced phytotoxic effect of the chemical presumably due to its lower initial availability to the plant.

Spring 1975 saw the installation of a second test. This evaluation was designed to determine the long-range effects of two controlled release formulations of Mocap, 10 and 25% microgranules. The pesticide was applied on March 15, 1974 and the plots immediately overplanted. Harvest took place in late May. A second crop was planted in August with harvest in mid-September. No reapplication of nematocide was made between the spring and fall seasons. The data in Table III show that both the 10 and 25% formulations were effective in controlling the target organism seven months as indicated by the root knot indices. Yields were reduced by the 25% composite during the spring season again because of the phytotoxicity of the chemical.

Table III

Long range effect of controlled release nematocides on the yield and on control of root-knot nematocides of cucumbers.

Treatment	Rate (lbs.AI/acre)	Yield (bu/acre)	Root-Knot Index	Yield (bu/acre)	Root-Knot Index
10% AI lignin composite	4	487	0	112	1
25% AI lignin composite	4	390	0	135	0
Check	0	432	0	125	3.5

Application date - March 15, 1975
First harvest - May 30, 1975
Replant date - August 2, 1975
Second harvest - September 12, 1975

Fall data reveal that the "higher loading" composite was more effective during the second half of the test both from a control and yield standpoint.

Aside from control of nematodes which account for millions of dollars in losses annually (8) to growers of field crops, fruit and nuts, and vegetable crops, protection of crops from the effect of the very chemical designed to protect them from the microscopic worms has been shown to be a very desirable side effect of controlled release formulations. Fall 1976 provided an additional opportunity to study this phenomenon. A very wet and cool growing season eliminated nematode activity so a test was run simply to study yield effects. Table IV contains the data which is self-explanatory.

Table IV
Effect of controlled release and conventional nematocides on the yield of cucumbers. Fall 1976.

Treatment	Rate (lbs.AI/acre)	Yield (bu/acre)
25% EI Mocap/lignin	4 lbs.	247
10% AI Mocap/lignin	4 lbs.	263
Mocap 10G	4 lbs.	205
Fumazone 86E	½ gal.	187
Control	0	305

Lignin - PCNB.

The third system to be studied was a technical kraft lignin - Terraclor (PCNB) system prepared by coprecipitating the fungicide with the lignin from an aqueous solution. Field work was done at the Delta Experiment Station in Stoneville, Mississippi under the direction of C. P. Hegwood. The test organism was the soil fungus Rhizoctonia Solani responsible for "fruit rot" of cucumbers, tomatoes, and peanuts. This particular organism is responsible for excessive crop losses in areas where it infects the soil. For example, during 1976, over 50% of the cucumbers grown on the Mississippi Delta, for processing into pickles were discarded (9) inflicting economic losses to growers. Processor tomatoes cannot be grown in the same area because of problems associated with R. solani despite near perfect climatic conditions.(10)

Following a spring 1976 field test where the lignin/PCNB composite, a 50% wettable powder, was identified along with several conventional formulations, as being effective in controlling the microorganisms, a series of greenhouse tests were instituted.

Soil samples from the same field used in the spring tests were sterilized and placed in aluminum pans. R. solani inoculum was placed on all of the soil samples and allowed to incubate. Fungicides were then applied to the pans at rates recommended by their respective manufacturers. Subsequently, fresh cucumbers were placed on the soils, covered with a polyethylene sheet, and allowed to remain undisturbed for five days. Following this, the fruit was removed from the pans and examined for fruit rot lesions.

Date in Table V describes the results of the work.

Table V
Fungicide Screening Data - Single Application
Percentage of Infected Fruit

Treatment	Days After Application 11	17	24	49
PC-474*	42	0	25	8
PC-460**	17	8	33	8
Terraclor	8	0	42	45
Terraclor (Tech.)	58	25	67	83
Nabac	100	92	100	83
Nabac (Tech)	100	100	100	92
Difolatan	92	100	83	75
Lignin	100	100	100	100
Check	100	100	100	100

* 60% wettable powder containing 19% of its active content as free un-incorporated PCNB.

** 50% wettable powder containing 100% of its active content as incorporated PCNB.

Seven weeks after application, the two lignin based formulations were still effective in keeping the microorganisms under control. This is somewhat significant since current practive involves fungicide application shortly after planting with repeated application at weekly intervals. Such costly procedures continue until the plants reach a layby stage. Here the plants form a dense canopy and shield the ground with their foliage. At this time conventional fungicides cannot be successfully applied to the ground or the fruit and foliage of the plants. From this point on, the ripening fruit must depend upon residual fungicide for protection. The time elapsed between planting and harvest for processor type cucumbers is 45-50 days.

A system such as PC-460 or PC-474 which remains effective for six or seven weeks would make it possible for the grower to rely on a single application of fungicide at the time of planting and at the same time realize yields, if not unmarked, at least less severely scarred by losses due to fruit rot.

Conclusions

The three systems evaluated thus far demonstrate the feasibility of the use of kraft lignin as a controlled release carrier system. Modifications of kraft lignin can also be used as carriers to extend the period of biological activity of pesticides, reduce their application rates, and reduce the frequency of application in cases where the parent lignin cannot be used.

Acknowledgement

The author wishes to express his gratitude to Dr. Wayne Sitterly of the Clemson University Truck Experiment Station, Charleston, S. C. and Dr. C. P. Hegwood of the Delta Experiment Station, Stoneville, Mississippi for the field evaluation of the nematocide and fungicide composites and to Dr. S. I. Falkehag and Mr. H. H. Moorer of the Westvaco Corporation for their encouragement and guidance of this work.

Literature Cited

(1) Nimz, H., Angew Chem. Internat, Ed., 13 313 (1974).
(2) Lindberg, J. J., Tylli, H., and Magani, C., Paperi Puu, 46, 521 (1964).
(3) Rezanowich, A., Yean, W. Q., and Goring, D. A. I., Svensk Papperstidn., 66, 141 (1963).
(4) Gupta, P. R., and Goring, D. A. I., Can. J. Chem., 38, 270 (1960).
(5) Marton, J., and Marton, T., Tappi, 47, 471 (1964).
(6) Christman, R. F., and Oglesby, R. T. in Lignin, Occurrances and Structures, Sarkanen and Ludwig, Editors Wiley New York (1971).
(7) Small, P. A., J. Appl. Chem., 3, (Feb., 1953).
(8) Feldmeser, J., USDA-ARS Beltsville, Md., Private Communication.
(9) Hegwood, C. P., Delta Experiment Station, Private Communication.
(10) Batson, W. E., Mississippi State University, Private Communication.

9

Controlled Release of Herbicides from Biodegradable Substrates

G. G. ALLAN,* J. W. BEER, and N. J. COUSIN

College of Forest Resources, University of Washington, Seattle, Wash. 98195

The controlled release concept now seems to have gained a firm foothold in pesticide technology as evidenced by the plethora of symposia which have been organized around the U.S. in recent years (1-3).

Although many different controlled release techniques have been presented at these gatherings actually few have progressed beyond laboratory evaluation. Among those which have is a controlled release herbicide primarily intended as a reforestation aid (4). This is based on the chemical linkage of a herbicide to a biodegradable substrate by means of a hydrolyzable bond. After this chemical combination is placed on the forest floor, herbicide is slowly released to suppress the growth of competitive vegetation in the vicinity of the seedling for a period of time, measured in months or years.

However, if this type of controlled release herbicide which has been successful in forestry is to be used in agriculture shorter periods of release will be more appropriate.

The design of such systems is now underway and this paper describes an assessment of the effect of the degree of substitution on the rate of hydrolytic degradation of α-cellulose 2,4-dichlorophenoxyacetate both *in vitro* and *in vivo*.

Results and Discussion

The α-cellulose 2,4-dichlorophenoxyacetates studied in this project contained 4.1, 4.9 or 21.5% by weight of combined herbicide. The rates of hydrolysis for these biocides in water at varying pH values are quite different. The data in Figure 1 shows that the release is dependent on both the degree of substitution and the acidity or alkalinity of the hydrolysis medium. Moreover, since the hydrolysis samples contained the same quantity of combined active ingredient it is clear that a faster release of

*Address inquiries to Professor G. G. Allan, University of Washington, AR-10, Seattle, WA 98195.

herbicide was obtained with the α-cellulose ester having the lower degree of substitution. This pattern of herbicide release can be explained in terms of the micro-structure of the α-cellulose fiber which contains dispersed crystalline (60%) and amorphous (40%) regions. In nonpolar nonswelling reaction media the latter provides essentially all of the readily available reactive hydroxy groups. In unswollen native cellulose those amount to only 0.4% of the total fiber material (5). This value is increased to 0.54% as a result of the isolation procedures which generate about one third more surface area (6). Thus, it can be anticipated that esterification reactions will begin randomly on accessible amorphous surfaces and subsequently spread along the polysaccharide chains. As a result, the density and pattern of substituents will vary throughout the α-cellulose substrate (I). This variance is compounded by the unequal reactivities of the hydroxy groups on each anhydroglucose unit towards esterification. For example, tosylation experiments have shown that the C_6, C_2 and C_3 hydroxy groups are esterified in the ratio of 215:33:1 respectively (7). Furthermore, a kinetic study demonstrated that the primary hydroxy group reacts fifty-eight times faster than its secondary neighbors (8).

As a result of all these facts, it can be concluded that esterification reactions of α-cellulose at low degrees of substitution will randomly occur almost exclusively on the fiber surfaces associated with the amorphous region at the primary hydroxy groups of the C_6 carbon atom of each glucose unit. It therefore follows that in the α-cellulose derivative there will be groups of more or less closely located ester units separated by areas having only an occasional ester substituent and hence a hydrophilic character comparable to the original amorphous region of the α-cellulose. Of course, as the degree of substitution is increased, the size of these hydrophilic areas must decrease. Ultimately, the hydrophilicity can become so small that water cannot permeate the polymer matrix (9) to effect hydrolytic release of the herbicide (10, 11).

This structural picture therefore provides a satisfying explanation for hydrolytic release data in Figure 1 since the more hydrophilic α-cellulose ester can be expected to hydrolyze at a faster rate than the more hydrophobic polymeric ester. Obviously a defining minimum limit must exist where further decreases in the amount of pendant ester linkages will not lead to a faster rate of hydrolysis. This level remains to be established.

In spite of the clarity of these hydrolytic experiments, the actual behavior of the α-cellulose ester in soil will be somewhat more complex. Certainly hydrolytic cleavage of the pendant ester will occur in the soil but this scission will be supplemented by microbial and enzymic attack on the α-cellulose derivative. It is well known (12) that rapid deterioration of cellulose occurs in soil and that the tensile properties of regenerated rayon, for example, are completely lost after fourteen days of soil burial.

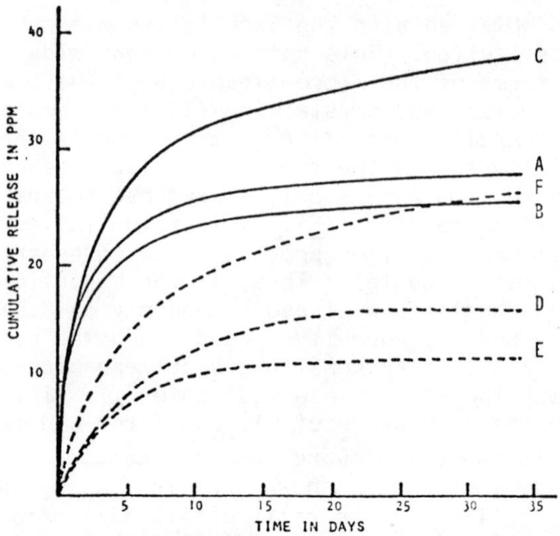

Figure 1. The cumulative release of 2,4-D from its α-cellulose esters where A, B, *and* C *are the 4.1% w/w combinations exposed to solutions of pH 4, 7, and 10, respectively, and* D, E, *and* F *are the corresponding treatments of the 21.5% w/w combinations subjected to the same treatments*

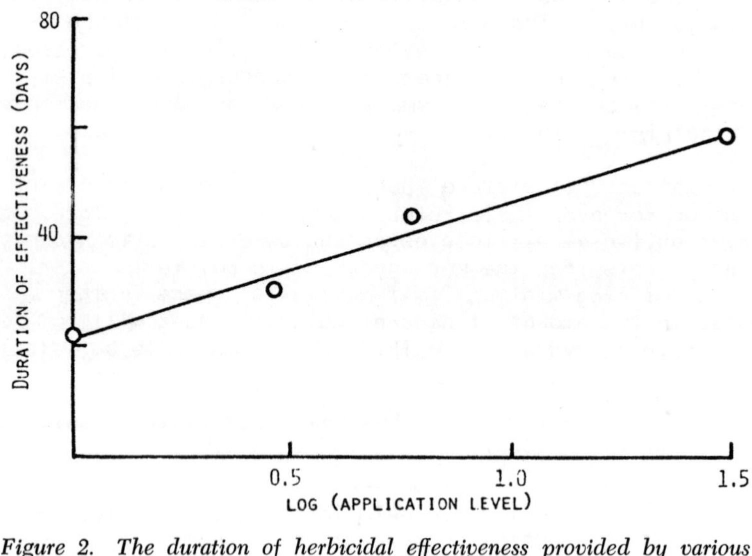

Figure 2. The duration of herbicidal effectiveness provided by various application levels of α-cellulose 2,4-dichlorophenoxyacetate (D.S. 0.05)

However, the α-cellulose release matrix need not be destroyed within this short period of time because of the protective effect of the esterifying herbicide acid. Thus, in contrast to the unesterified cellulose fibers, the physical properties of their monoacetylated counterparts were not adversely affected by exposure to soil burial for six months (13).

These enzymic and microbial parameters can best be explored under actual use conditions, that is, by experiments using soil. However, to obtain reproducible results in a bioassay it is necessary to carefully control the conditions. Under such precise conditions the rate of surface hydrolysis for an ester of a water insoluble polymer in a moisture inundated soil can be written as

$$-dC/dt = KC \tag{1}$$

where C is the concentration of the herbicide per unit weight of the α-cellulose ester at time t and K is the degradation rate constant. When C_o is the value of C at time zero then, separation of the variables in equation I, and integration affords the relationship

$$C = C_o e^{-Kt} \tag{2}$$

At the critical time t_c which marks the end of the period of herbicidal effectiveness of the α-cellulose ester, the rate of release R for an application of weight W follows from equation (2) so that

$$R = WKC_o e^{-Kt_c} \tag{3}$$

Since the time to reach this critical point is actually the duration of herbicidal effectiveness (D_{pr}) then

$$D_{pr} = M \log W - N \tag{4}$$

where M = 2.3/K and N = (2.3/K)log(R/C_oK). Therefore, a plot of the duration of herbicidal effectiveness versus the logarithm of the weight of α-cellulose 2,4-dichlorophenoxyacetate applied should give a straight line (10). Although the data in Fig. 2 validates equation 4 it must be remembered that these soil experiments are very well controlled. Under the uncontrolled conditions of actual use the pattern of release will be much more complex. As an illustration, Figure 3 shows the complex climatological data for a field site in the Sedro Woolley area of Washington where a controlled release herbicide test was carried out.

Obviously, the high temperatures of midyear would be expected to kinetically accelerate the rate of hydrolysis of α-cellulose esters. However, in actual fact, the lack of water at this time probably means that the rate of hydrolysis will be minimal. Conversely, the abundant moisture available at the beginning and end of the year, which would facilitate hydrolysis, is counterbalanced by the freezing temperatures which will slow the rate of hydrolysis. This type of climate-modified rate of release is unique to chemically bonded systems and constitutes a strong rationale for the initial selection of this type of controlled release system. In contrast, encapsulation or other diffusion-controlled processes will not turn themselves off when temperature rise and moisture levels fall. Indeed, release from such devices actually will speed up under conditions which are already generally unfavorable for the germination of the weeds to be controlled. Clearly, this is intrinsically wasteful and inefficient.

Therefore, although bioassays are more informative than hydrolysis, actual field performance is the final and superior arbiter. However, controlled laboratory bioassays in soil can provide useful preliminary guidance in the design of controlled release herbicides and in this type of test the free herbicide inhibited germination for nine days as depicted in Figure 4. The controlled release α-cellulose derivatives containing the same amount of herbicide as was applied in the free state lasted 30% and 100% longer. The relatively small differences in the length of the period of effectiveness is due to the fact that the α-cellulose esters contain no free herbicide. That is, the herbicide released by hydrolysis is not functioning only to replace the losses from a pre-established effective level of free herbicide. Instead, in this demanding bioassay, the α-cellulose ester must first release enough herbicide to attain the minimum effective level and subsequently maintain this by additional hydrolysis. Obviously this stringent demand reduces the duration of the period of effectiveness. This explains the shorter period of effectiveness which is provided by the α-cellulose ester with the higher degree of substitution. That is, the lower rate of release of this derivative cannot maintain for long the required level of free herbicide for effective performance. Under field conditions this situation would be avoided by coadministration of the controlled release herbicide together with the small amount of free herbicide necessary to immediately attain in the soil the minimum effective level required to inhibit germination.

Of course, a practical controlled release herbicide system should not be designed in a vacuum. Among the many design factors which have to be taken in account, the duration of the period of effectiveness is one of the most important. The attainment of this specification can be manipulated most readily by variation of the level of esterification. This is generally the case irrespective of the substrate. Although the release rate does certainly depend on the chemical structure of the substrate (14) the effect of changing substrates is minor relative to the influence of the levels of herbicide combined with the polymer. That is, for a given substrate, as the degree of substitution is increased the rate of release of herbicide is sharply decreased. This concept cannot be extended indefinitely because at higher degrees of substitution the hydrophobicity will become so great that the

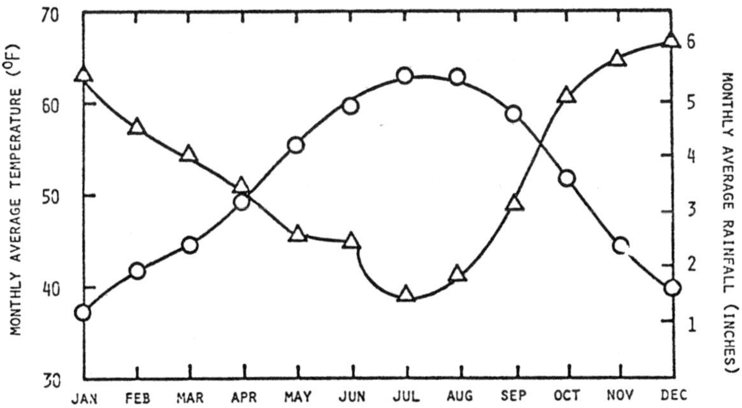

Figure 3. Monthly average temperature (○) and rainfall (△) for a forest plantation site near Sedro Woolley, Wash.

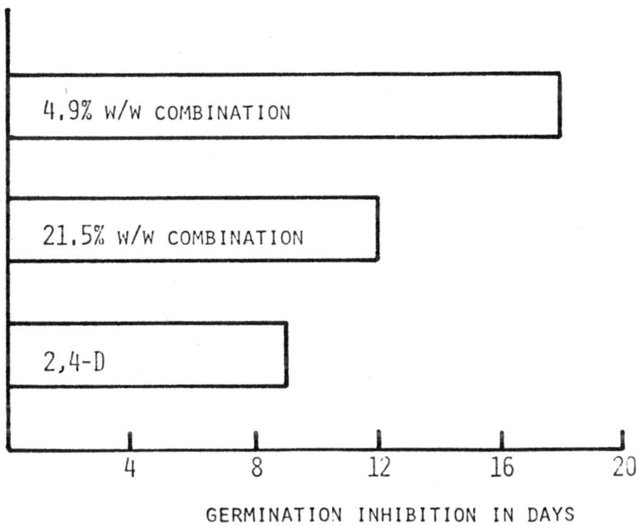

Figure 4. A comparison of the persistence of germination inhibition by bioassay between two different w/w-controlled release combinations of α-cellulose 2,4-dichlorophenoxyacetate and the active herbicide at 0.68 mg A.I./cm²

polymeric ester will become essentially nonhydrolyzable. On the other hand, the supermolecular structure is relatively unimportant as long as there are sufficient amorphous regions to attain a reasonable level of active herbicide in the α-cellulose ester. In practice, formulations containing 10 or 20% active ingredient are the most compatible with existing application equipment and techniques. The existence of all these release parameters provides such a flexibility of design that it can be confidently anticipated that controlled release herbicides based on chemical linkages to biodegradable substrates will be an important part of this emergent area of pesticide technology.

Experimental

Esterification of α-cellulose with 2,4-dichlorophenoxyacetic acid. A suspension of oven-dried (105°C) α-cellulose fibers (50g) in anhydrous benzene (200ml) at 22° was treated portion-wise (2ml) with a solution of 2,4-dichlorophenoxyacetyl chloride (8.7 or 24.0g) in anhydrous benzene (50ml) and refluxed. After 3 h the reaction mixture was evaporated to near dryness and filtered. The residue was exhaustively extracted (Soxhlet) with benzene, washed with water, air and oven-dried before ball-milling to afford α-cellulose 2,4-dichlorophenoxyacetate as a fine powder. The extent of esterification (4.1, 4.9 and 21.5% w/w) was calculated from chlorine analysis of the products using the neutron activation technique of irradiating samples in a neutron flux (1.4×10^{11} neutron/cm^2 sec) for 10 min. After appropriate cooling, the samples were counted by integrating the 1.33 MeV photopeak of ^{38}Cl with 2.27 KeV (FWHM) using a Ge(Li) crystal and a multichannel analyzer. The Ge(Li) crystal (Princeton Gamma-Tech) had an efficiency rating of 10.6% relative to a NaI (Tℓ) 3x3 in. crystal and was located 25 cm from the source.

Hydrolytic release of 2,4-dichlorophenoxyacetic acid from α-cellulose 2,4-dichlorophenoxyacetate. Triplicate samples of α-cellulose 2,4-dichlorophenoxyacetate (DS 0.03 and 0.16) sized to contain 125mg of releasable 2,4-dichlorophenoxyacetic acid, were enveloped in four layers of porous teabag paper ("Flo-Thru^R, Thomas J. Lipton, Inc., Englewood Cliffs, NJ) which when sealed had an outer surface area of $50cm^2$. These bags were then suspended in unstirred distilled water (500ml), adjusted to pH values of 4, 7 and 10 using NaOH or HCl, and maintained at a temperature of 22°. Thereafter, at various elapsed times the bags were removed and resuspended in freshly prepared solutions while the residual solutions were analyzed for their content of 2,4-dichlorophenoxyacetic acid using a Dohrmann Environtech DC-50 Total Organic Carbon Analyzer.

Bioassay of the duration of herbicidal effectiveness of α-cellulose 2,4-dichlorophenoxyacetate. Quadruplicate mixtures (1g) of α-cellulose 2,4-dichlorophenoxyacetate (containing 31.1mg of combined 2,4-dichlorophenoxyacetic acid) and oven-dried (105°)

sized (40-60 mesh, U.S. Standard Sieve Series) soil were evenly spread over the surface of nonsterile composted soil (7x7x5cm) contained in rectangular plastic pots. Controls containing zero or free herbicide were similarly prepared. Ten cucumber seeds (Petoseed SMR 18, Variety 051, thiram treated, Petoseed Co., Inc., Satuoy, CA) were presoaked in water for 2h and randomly placed on the soil surface of each pot which was then covered with a clear plastic petri dish. All treatment replicates were placed together in separate water-filled aluminum trays (26.7x39.4x2.5cm) in a controlled environment room (constant light at 21° and 65% relative humidity). Thereafter each 3 days the germinated root structures were compared to those of the controls (1-1.5cm root length; mycorhiza present). The seedlings and the ungerminated seeds were then removed and replaced with freshly presoaked seeds. The standing water in the aluminum tray was also replaced at this time. This entire procedure was repeated until the number of the germinating seeds in the pots containing the α-cellulose 2,4-dichlorophenoxyacetate were statistically equivalent to those in the control.

Literature Cited

1. Allan, G.G. and Noogi, A.N., in Controlled Release of Biologically Active Agents, Eds., A.C. Tanquary and R.E. Lacey, Plenum Press, NY, 1974, 195.
2. Harris, F.W., Proceedings International Controlled Release Pesticide Symposium, College of Science and Engineering, Wright State University, Dayton, Ohio, 1975.
3. Cardarelli, N.F., Controlled Release Pesticide Symposium, Engineering and Science Division, Community and Technical College, The University of Akron, Akron, Ohio, 1976.
4. Allan, G.G., Friedhoff, J.F. and Powell, J.C., Intern. Pest Control, 1974, 12 (2), 4.
5. Timell, T., Ph.D. Thesis, Royal Institute of Technology, Stockholm, Sweden, 1960.
6. Jörgensen, L. and Ribi, E., Nature, 1950, 166, 148.
7. Gardner, T.S. and Purves, C.B., J. Am. Chem. Soc., 1942, 64, 1539.
8. Honeyman, J., J. Chem. Soc., 1947, 168.
9. Higuchi, T. and Aguar, A., J. Pharm. Sci., 1959, 45, 578.
10. Neogi, A.N., Ph.D. Thesis, University of Washington, Seattle, Washington, 1970.
11. Wilkins, R.M., M.S. Thesis, University of Washington, Seattle, Washington, 1970.
12. Allan, F.J., Allan, G.G., Crank, G. and Thomson, J.B., J. Appl. Chem., 1962, 12, 46.
13. Buras, Jr., E.M., Cooper, A.S., Keating, E.J., and Goldthwait, C.F., Amer. Dyestuff Rep., 1954, 43, 203.
14. Allan, G.G., Belgian Patent 706,509 (1966); Australian Patent 423,990 (1967); Italian Patent 820,813 (1967); French Patent 1,544,406 (1968); Japanese Patent 558,788 (1969); U.K. Patent 1,212,842 (1970); Canadian Patents 855,181 (1970), 863,310 (1971); U.S. Patent 3,813,236 (1974).

10

Polymers Containing Pendant Herbicide Substituents: Hydrolysis Studies II

FRANK W. HARRIS, MARY R. DYKES, JIM A. BAKER, and ANN E. AULABAUGH

Department of Chemistry, Wright State University, Dayton, Ohio 45431

The objective of this research has been the development of controlled-release herbicides that will afford extended control of aquatic weeds (1,2). One approach to these materials has been the synthesis of polymers that contain herbicides as pendent substituents (3-5). For example, homopolymers have been prepared that consist of over 80% 2,4-dichlorophenoxyacetic acid (2,4-D) or 2-(2,4,5-trichlorophenoxy)propionic acid (Silvex) as pendent side chains. It was postulated that the herbicide would be released from these systems by the slow, sequential hydrolysis of the herbicide-polymer bonds. Hydrolysis studies, however, showed that the homopolymers will not undergo hydrolysis under mildly alkaline conditions at 30° (6).

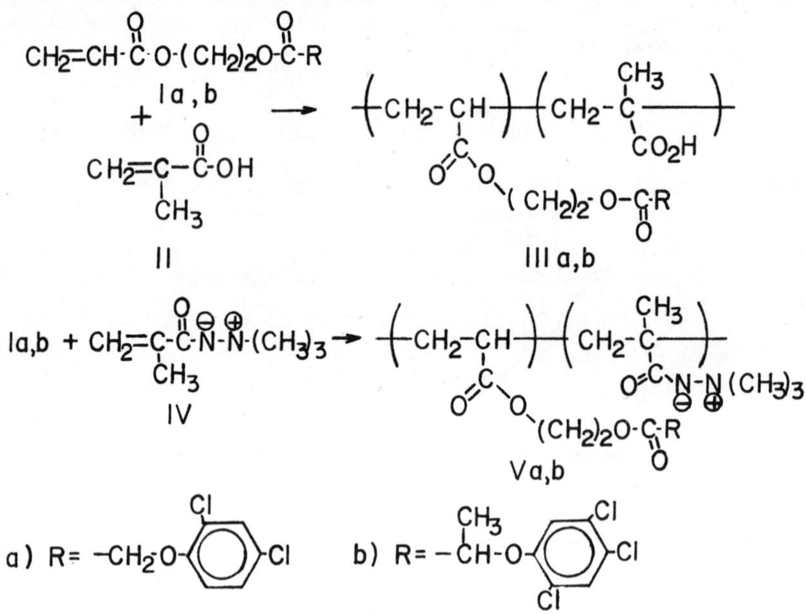

The reactivity of substituents attached to the backbone of a polymer chain is known to be substantially increased by the presence of suitable neighboring groups (7). For example, the hydrolysis of pendent ester groups is enhanced by the incorporation of carboxyl groups along the backbone (8-11). In an attempt to similarly facilitate the hydrolysis of herbicide-polymer bonds, copolymers were prepared that contained pendent herbicide esters and carboxyl groups. Copolymers containing herbicides and hydrophilic aminimide residues were also prepared. Thus, the copolymerization of the 2-acryloyloxyethyl esters of 2,4-D (Ia) and Silvex (Ib) with methacrylic acid (II) and trimethylamine methacrylimide (IV) afforded the polymers III and V. A preliminary hydrolysis study of polymer IIIa containing 20 mole percent methacrylic acid indicated that the copolymer undergoes relatively rapid hydrolysis at pH 8 and 30°. (A 1-g sample of the copolymer released 117 mg of 2,4-D in the first 6 days of the study.) Copolymers containing the aminimide residue, however, hydrolyzed slowly under these conditions. (A 1-g sample of Va containing 35 mole percent IV released 18 mg of 2,4-D in 32 days.) Decreasing the percentage of IV in Copolymer Va resulted in a decrease in the rate of hydrolysis (6).

This communication describes the preparation and subsequent hydrolyses of samples of copolymer IIIa which contain reduced amounts of methacrylic acid. The final results of the study of the hydrolysis of copolymer Va are also presented. In addition, a copolymer of 2-methacryloyloxyethyl 2,4-dichlorophenoxyacetate and methacrylic acid has been prepared and subjected to mild hydrolysis conditions.

Results and Discussion

Copolymers of 2-Acryloyloxyethyl 2,4-Dichlorophenoxyacetate and Methacrylic Acid. The 2-acryloyloxyethyl ester of 2,4-D (Ia) was copolymerized with 5 and 10 mole per cent methacrylic acid (II), i.e. the molar feed ratios of Ia:II used were 95:5 and 90:10, respectively. The polymerizations were carried out in 2-butanone with azobisisobutyronitrile (AIBN) as the initiator to afford 80-82% yields of the white products. The copolymers are soluble in chlorinated hydrocarbons and have inherent viscosities of 0.12 and 0.14 (0.5 g/dl in 2-butanone at 30°), respectively.

Three samples of each copolymer were immersed in a buffered aqueous solution that was maintained at 30°. A pH of 8 was used to simulate the pH of the natural waters in the South where the aquatic weed problems are the most pronounced. The amount of herbicide released from the samples was determined periodically by spectrophotometric analysis. A plot of the average amount of 2,4-D released from the three replicates of each copolymer with time is shown in Figure 1. The hydrolyses were accompanied by considerable swelling of the polymer

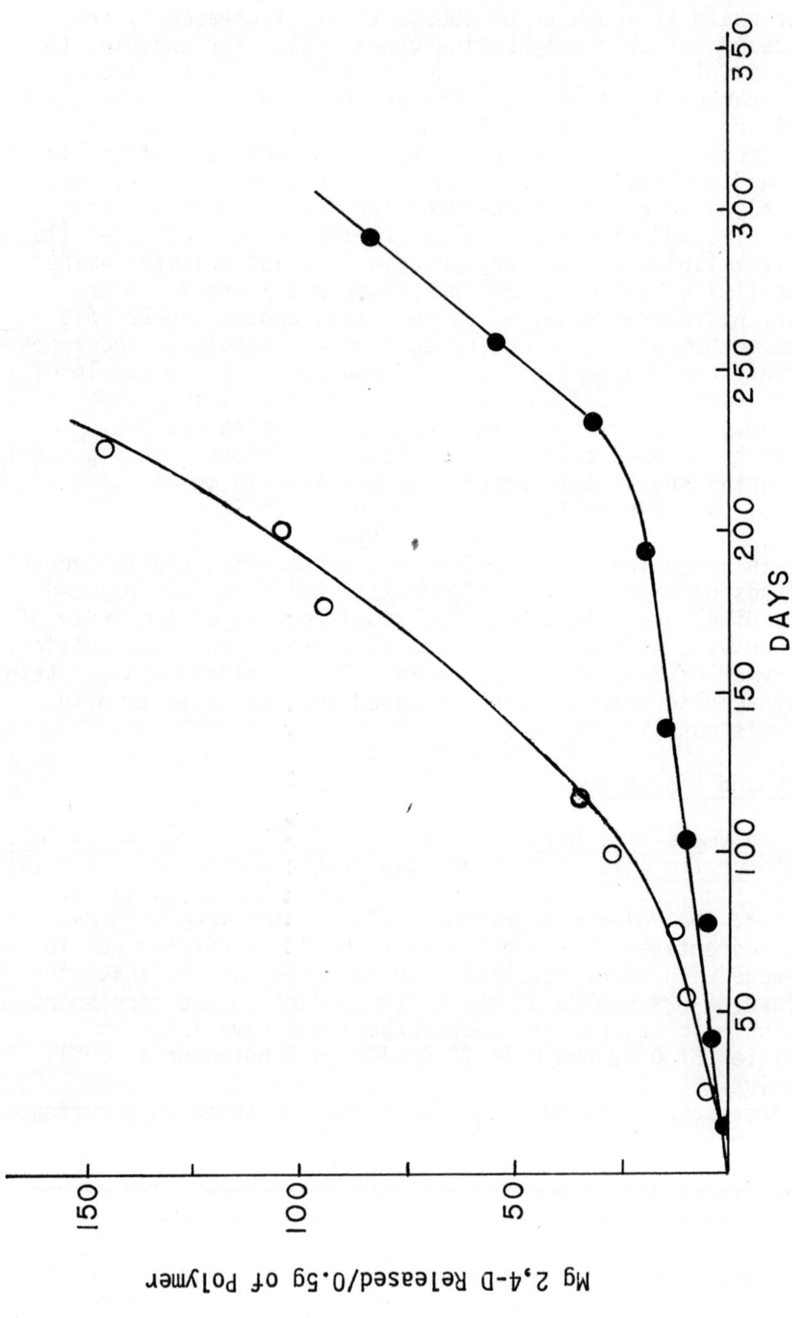

Figure 1. Hydrolysis of methacrylic acid copolymers. (○) *90:10 copolymer of 2-acryloyloxyethyl 2,4-dichlorophenoxyacetate and methacrylic acid.* (●) *95:5 copolymer of 2-acryloyloxyethyl 2,4-dichlorophenoxyacetate and methacrylic acid.*

particles, which eventually prevented further spectroscopic analysis of the solutions. In fact, the last point on the hydrolysis curve of the 90:10 2-acryoyloxyethyl 2,4-dichlorophenoxyacetate: methacrylic acid copolymer may be high due to the cloudiness of the analytical samples. One of the replicates of this copolymer was acidified and extracted with ether after 296 days. Approximately 290 mg of pure 2,4-D, which represents 87% of the 2,4-D originally contained in the polymer, was recovered.

As can be seen in Figure 1, the rate of hydrolysis of both copolymers increased with time. This is similar to the autoacceleration in rate observed in the hydrolysis of polyacrylamides (12) and poly(vinyl acetate) (13). In these cases, the acceleration has been ascribed to intramolecular interactions of neighboring groups generated during the hydrolyses. The rapid hydrolysis of ester groups incorporated along a poly(acrylic acid) chain has also been attributed to a neighboring group effect (8). The enhanced hydrolysis is thought to be due to an internal nucleophilic attack of a neighboring carboxylate ion on the carbonyl carbon of the ester group, with the formation of a

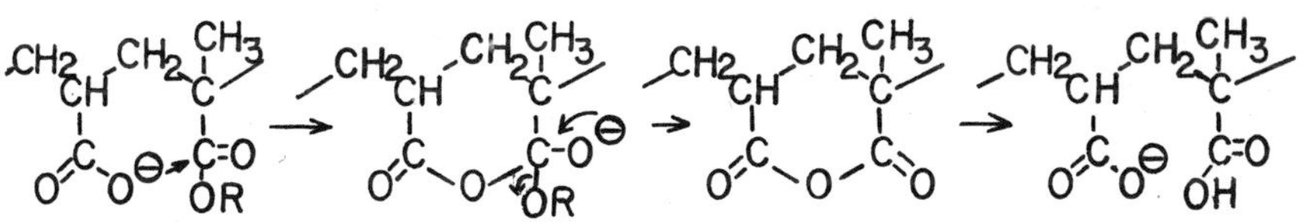

six-membered acid anhydride intermediate being rate determining. Considerable subsequent work has substantiated that intermolecular reactions are practically negligible in comparison to the intramolecular functional interactions between an ester group and a directly vicinal acid or carboxylate group. Steric hindrance, however, can reduce or prevent the neighboring group effect (14).

In the present study, the interaction of a neighboring carboxyl group should result in the generation of 2-hydroxyethyl 2,4-dichlororophenoxyacetate (VI). Nearly quantitative amounts of

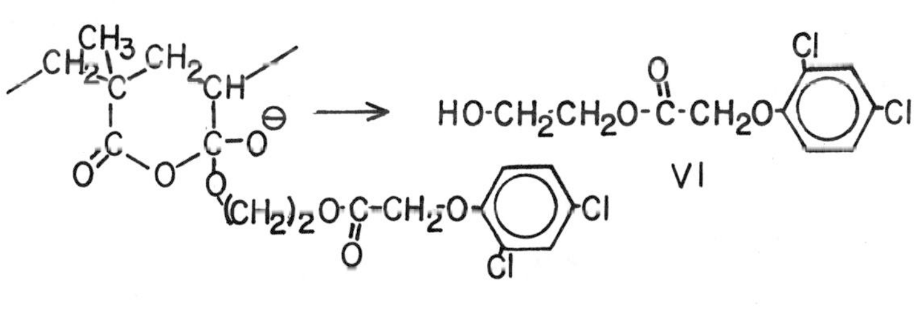

VI

pure 2,4-D, however have been extracted from the hydrolysis solutions. It is possible that compound VI undergoes subsequent hydrolysis to afford 2,4-D and ethylene glycol. Preliminary analyses of the sample solutions for ethylene glycol indicate that only 20 to 40% of the theoretical amount is present. The hydrolysis of compound VI at pH 8 is currently being investigated.

Another possible explanation for the acceleration in rate involves intramolecular interactions of carboxyl and ester groups that are not located on neighboring residues in the polymer chain. In this case, the rate of hydrolysis reflects the probability of chain conformations that bring the two interacting groups into juxtaposition and, hence, is related to chain flexibility and mobility. The enhanced hydrolysis of acrylamide terpolymers containing pendent ester and catalytic substituents has been shown to be due to such interactions (15). It has also been demonstrated that in order for the catalysis to occur the ester group must not be sterically hindered. Thus, ester groups that are located several atoms away from the terpolymer backbone hydrolyze rapidly while those attached directly to the backbone hydrolyze at the normal intermolecular rate.

The polymers in the present study underwent considerable swelling and gradual dissolution as the hydrolysis proceeded. Hence, the probability of intramolecular interactions between distant ester and carboxyl groups was increased. Due to steric effects, the carboxyl groups should only attack the 2,4-D ester

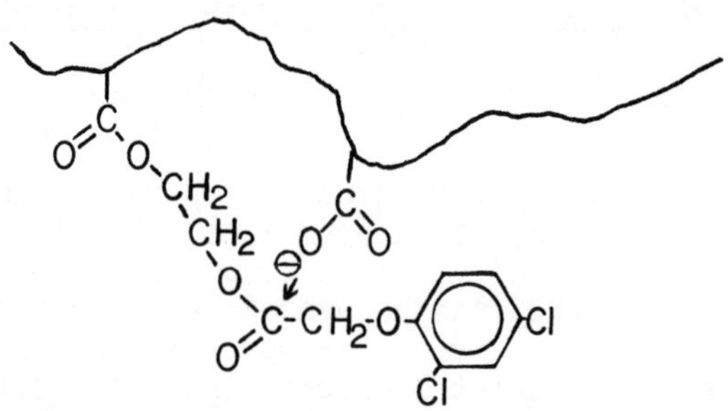

carbonyls, which would result in the release of pure 2,4-D. The presence of more 2,4-D than ethylene glycol in the hydrolysis mixtures indicates that considerable hydrolysis did occur at the 2,4-D-polymer ester bond. It is postulated that the initial hydrolysis of the copolymers is due to neighboring group interactions with subsequent hydrolysis resulting from the interactions of distant groups.

Copolymer of 2-Methacryloyloxyethyl 2,4-Dichlorophenoxyacetate and Methacrylic Acid. The 2-methacryloyloxyethyl ester of 2,4-D (VII) was prepared from 2,4-dichlorophenoxyacetyl chloride and 2-hydroxyethyl methacrylate by the previously described procedure (2). The copolymerization of this monomer with 10 mole percent methacrylic acid by the procedure described for the acrylic ester afforded a 65% yield of VIII. The white copolymer was soluble in chlorinated hydrocarbons and had an inherent viscosity of 0.14 (0.5 g/dl in 2-butanone at 30°).

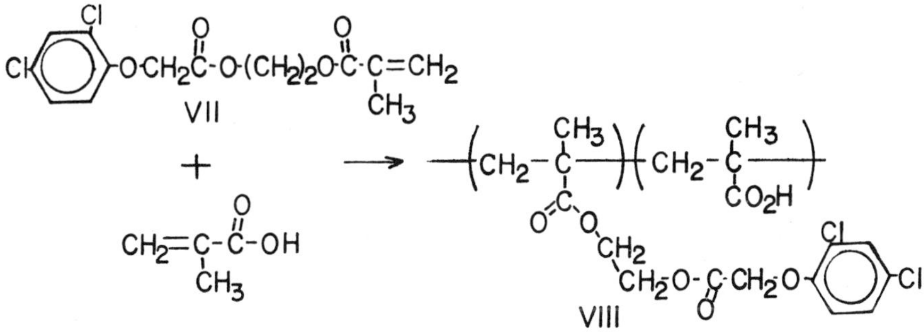

Samples of VIII were also immersed in a pH 8 buffer maintained at 30°. The copolymer, however, did not undergo hydrolysis under these mild conditions. This decrease in reactivity may be due to increased steric hindrance in the formation of the proposed cyclic-anhydride intermediate. In the methacrylic copolymers, the six-membered ring is tetrasubstituted in the 1,1' and 3,3' positions which results in considerable

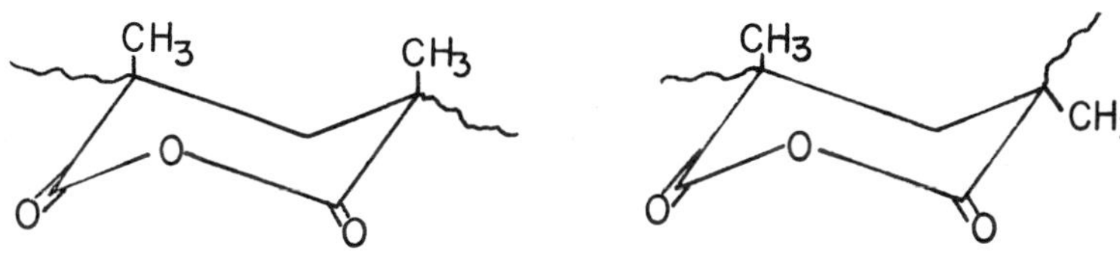

steric hindrance between the two axial substituents. This argument has been used to explain the fact that methacrylic acid-methyl methacrylate copolymers hydrolyze about 10-12 times more slowly at 110° than acrylic acid-methyl acrylate copolymers with the same molar composition (10).

Copolymer of 2-Acryloyloxyethyl 2,4-Dichlorophenoxyacetate and Trimethylamine Methacrylimide. The previously described study of the hydrolysis of copolymer Va containing 35 mole percent trimethylamine methacrylimide was completed (6). The data shown in Figure 2 were obtained by employing the procedures used with the methacrylic acid copolymers. The study was terminated after 394 days at which time the copolymer had released 250 mg of 2,4-D per 0.5-g sample, which corresponds to

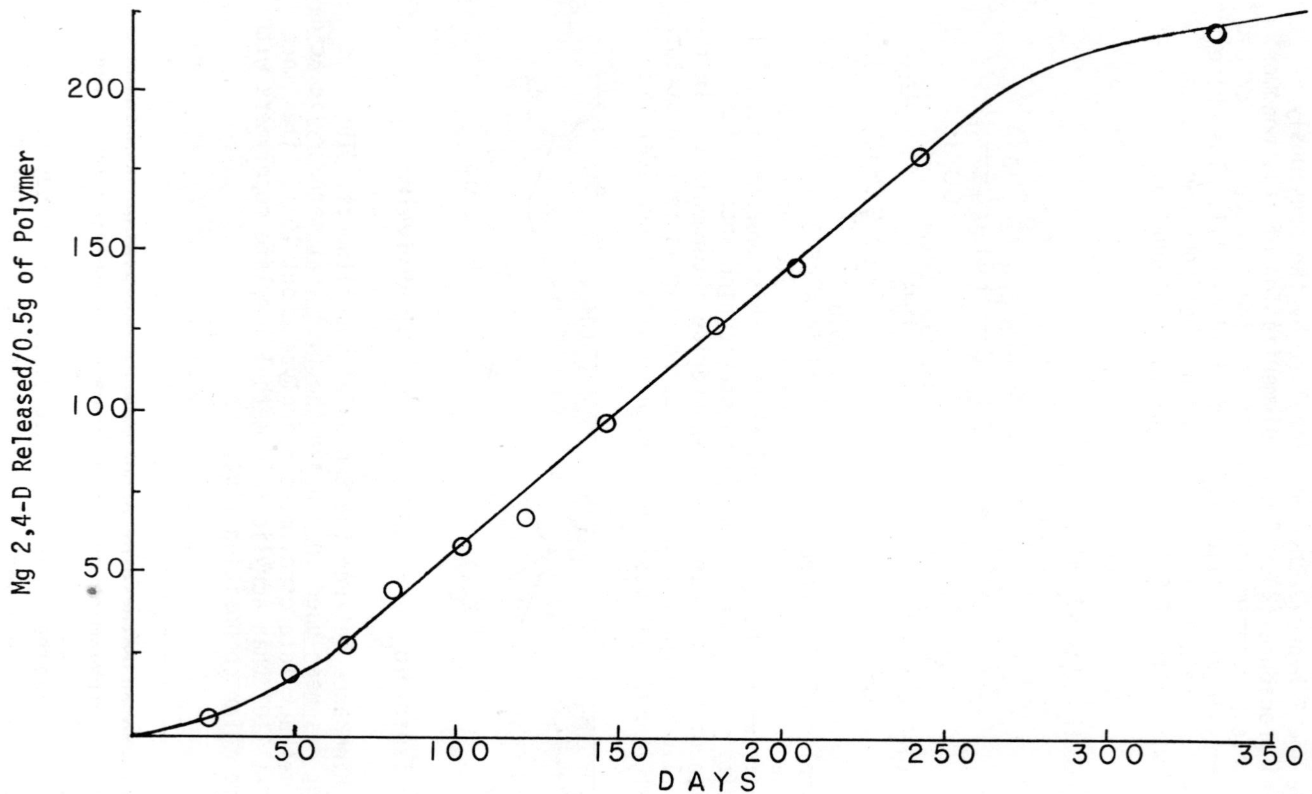

Figure 2. *Hydrolysis of trimethylamine methacrylimide copolymer.* (●) *65:35 copolymer of 2-acryloyloxyethyl 2,4-dichlorophenoxyacetate and trimethylamine methacrylimide.*

90% of the amount originally present. As can be seen from the Figure, the rate of hydrolysis increased during the first few days of the study and then remained relatively constant. Since the concentration of ester linkages decreases as the polymer is hydrolyzed, the rate constant for the hydrolysis must continually increase. This behavior, in effect, provides a zero-order rate of release, which is ideally suited for controlled-release applications.

The increase in the rate constant as the hydrolysis proceeds may also be due to intramolecular catalysis. Infrared data indicates that amine acylimides have a reasonance stabilized structure as shown (17). Hence, it is possible that the

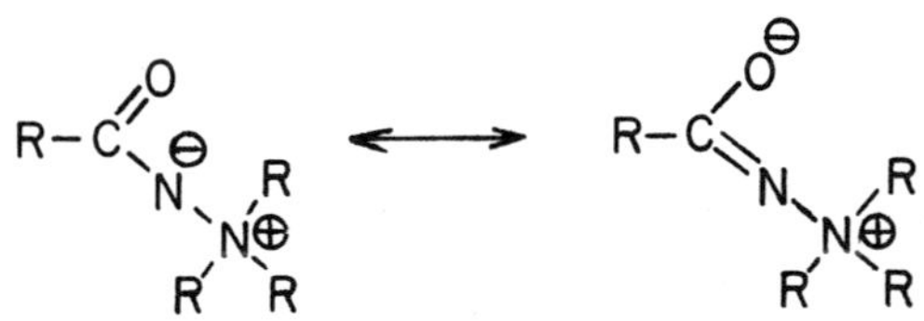

aminimide group acts as a catalyst in the same manner as described for the carboxyl group. The mechanism by which copolymer Va undergoes hydrolysis is currently being investigated.

Experimental

Ultraviolet spectra were obtained with a Cary Model 14 spectrophotometer. Infrared spectra were obtained on thin films with a Perkin-Elmer Model 457 spectrophotometer. Viscosities were determined with a Cannon Number 75 viscometer. The aminimide monomer was furnished by Ashland Chemicals, Columbus, Ohio.

General Solution Copolymerization Procedure. Herbicide monomer, comonomer, 2-butanone (4 ml/g of monomers), and 0.05% AIBN were thoroughly mixed and slowly heated under nitrogen to 75°. After heating at 75° for 3 hr, the mixture was cooled, diluted with 2-butanone, and precipitated in hexane. The copolymer was collected by filtration and dried under vacuum at 60° for 3 hr.

Hydrolysis Studies. The copolymers were extracted with ether for 18 hr to remove unreacted monomer, dried under vacuum, and then ground and sieved to a particle size of 125-400μ. Three 0.5-g samples of each copolymer were placed in 500-ml erlenmeyer flasks containing 300 ml of a boric acid-sodium hydroxide buffer (pH = 8.08). The flasks were maintained at 30 ± 0.1° in a constant temperature bath. The amount of herbicide released from each copolymer was determined periodically by spectrophotometric analysis at 198 nm.

Acknowledgement

Support of this research by the Department of the Army, U.S. Army Engineer Waterways Experiment Station under Contract DACW39-86-C-0016 (Neg.) is gratefully acknowledged. Appreciation is also expressed to AmChem Products, Inc. for furnishing the herbicides and to Ashland Chemicals Company for furnishing the aminimides used in this study.

Literature Cited

1. Harris, Frank W., Norris, Steve O., and Post, Larry K., Weed Science, (1973), 21 (4), 318.
2. Harris, Frank W. and Post, Larry K. in "Proceedings 1974 International Controlled Release Pesticide Symposium," Cardarelli, Nate F., Ed., The University of Akron, Ohio, 1974.
3. Harris, Frank W., and Post, Larry K., Am. Chem. Soc., Polym. Div., Preprints, (1975), 16 (2), 622.
4. Harris, Frank W. and Post, Larry K., J. Polym. Sci., Polymer Letters Ed., (1975), 13, 225.
5. Harris, Frank W., Feld, William A., and Bowen, Bonnie, in "Proceedings 1975 International Controlled Release Pesticide Symposium," p. 334 Harris, F.W., Ed., Wright State University, Dayton, Ohio, 1975.
6. Harris, Frank W., Aulabaugh, Ann E., Case, Robert D., Dykes, Mary K., and Feld, William A., "ACS Symposium Series, No. 33, Controlled-Release Polymeric Formulations," p. 222, Paul, D.R. and Harris, F.W., Ed., American Chemical Society, Washington, D.C., 1976.
7. Morawetz, H., "Macromolecules in Solution," pp. 422-426, Wiley, New York, 1965.
8. Morawetz, H., and Zimmering, P.E., J. Phys. Chem., (1954), 58, 753.
9. Gaetjens, E. and Morawetz, J. Amer. Chem. Soc., (1961), 83, 1738.
10. Morawetz, H., and Westhead, E.W., J. Polym. Sci., (1955), 16, 273.
11. VanBeylen, M.M. in "Stereochemistry of Macromolecules," Vol. 3, p. 335, Ketley, A.D., Ed., Marcel Dekker, New York, 1968.
12. Smets, G. and Hesbain, A.M., J. Polym. Sci., (1959), 40, 217.
13. Sakurada, I. and Sakaguchi, Y., Kobunshi Kagaku, (1956), 13, 441; Chem. Abst., (1957), 51, 17365 g.
14. Smets, G. and VanHumbeeck, W., J. Polym. Sci., (1963), 1, 1227.

15. Goodman, N. and Morawetz, H., J. Polym. Sci., Part C, (1970), 31, 177.
16. Smets, G., and DeLoecker, W., J. Polym. Sci., (1960), 45, 461.
17. McKillip, W.J., Sedor, E.A., Culbertson, B.M., and Wawzonek, S., Chem. Rev., (1973), 73, 255.

11

Synthesis, Characterization, and Release Mechanisms of Polymers Containing Pendant Herbicides

CHARLES L. McCORMICK and MICHAEL FOOLADI

Department of Polymer Science, University of Southern Mississippi, Hattiesburg, Miss. 39401

As the world's population rapidly increases, agriculture is faced with the demand for enhanced production utilizing chemicals with little or no detrimental effect on the surrounding environment. Pesticide leaching into drainage waters and subsequent transport into non-target areas is of growing ecological concern. The immensity of the problem is apparent when considering the total agricultural pesticide application and the annual run-off for drainage areas.

The Mississippi Watershed area alone covers 1,244,000 square miles including vast stretches of central U.S. farmland. The annual water discharge at the mouth of the Mississippi has been estimated to 7.8×10^{11} yds^3 and 2,000,000 tons of sediment are carried into the sea per day. The average annual rainfall over this area is about 30 inches, of which about one-fourth travels to the Gulf of Mexico by way of the Mississippi River (1,2).

In 1974, nearly 1.4 billion pounds of organic pesticides were sold by U.S. companies, representing a growth of 12% over 1973. Insecticides accounted for 50.4% of the total volume with the balance consisting of herbicides, fungicides, and plant hormones (3). With some pesticide systems, 70 - 80% of the useful chemical activity is lost by various mechanisms including interaction with non-target organisms. Scientists have measured the rates of loss of activity of various chemicals in terms of "persistence" levels. Persistent pesticides have been attacked in environmental studies due to their usual migration to non-target areas. However, it should be pointed out that some degree of persistence is necessary to yield weed, insect or fungus control for a reasonable period of time in the target area. Often the most persistent chemicals are also the most effective.

Several factors are known to determine persistence in the soil. These include (a) uptake and degradation by microorganisms, (b) loss through physical processes of volatilization and leaching, and (c) chemical changes such as photo-decomposition and chemical reactions (4).

The Environmental Protection Agency is imposing stringent requirements on several effective and previously widely used pesticides. The type, amount applied, specificity, and persistence of each pesticide will be under continuing scrutiny. The pest control agents must not merely control target organisms but must be harmless to humans, livestock, crops, fish, wildlife, beneficial insects, soil microorganisms, etc.

Dramatic improvements in analytical instrumentation have allowed claims of detection of trace amounts of organic chemicals in non-target areas in the parts per billion range. This advance, in conjunction with the controversy generated by adverse publicity on insecticides such as DDT and Mirex, has led to a flurry of experiments on nearly every chemical manufactured in the U.S. Particular emphasis has been placed on chemicals having potential impact on the aquatic environment. For example, Butler (5-12) has reported growing evidence that "the continuing use of pesticide chemicals is producing environmental changes or residues in the food web that may cause reproductive failure. ." Some organisms have been shown to accumulate or concentrate certain persistent pesticides at alarming rates. The oyster, for example, when continuously exposed to 0.1 ppb of DDT, was reported to concentrate in its tissues up to 7.0 ppm in a month. It may be predicted that chlorinated herbicides will soon come under attack (13, 28-30).

Stringent rules and regulations (apparently subject to frequent modification) have been imposed on agricultural chemical producers and consumers as a result of environmental studies. Many knowledgeable sources predict an impending disaster for the whole agricultural industry from the high costs of licensing, registration, and production of new pesticides. In 1976, new pesticide commercialization required an average of 2.5 years of research and development at a cost of over $10,000,000.00. The agricultural industry has, in general, responded to the environmental regulations by producing less persistant but often less effective pesticides, requiring more frequent application over an extended growing season. A more logical and certainly more fruitful approach is to attack the undesired "leaching" or transport of a given pesticide rather than its "persistence."

Agricultural chemical leaching and subsequent pesticide transport to non-target environments can be greatly reduced, possibly eliminated, by controlled-release systems based on macromolecules. Polymers can be synthesized which contain reactive chemical bonds to common pesticides; these bonds are subject to enzymatic or hydrolytic break-down at a controllable rate. The macromolecular nature of these systems will prevent dissolution, leaching and transport to non-target areas. Controlled-release can also reduce the number of applications and the quantity of chemical required for pest control. A number of naturally occurring polymers (25-27) offer excellent potential as raw materials for substrate preparation of controlled release systems. In addition, certain polysaccharides decompose yielding products beneficial to the soil.

Development of a commercial herbicide system must combine effectiveness, favorable economics, with little adverse environmental impact. The chemical must: (1) control weeds at reasonable dosages, (2) selectively control target organisms only, leaving beneficial insects, plants, and humans unharmed, (3) persist for a reasonable time, (4) be inexpensive for large scale usage, and (5) and be easily applied, (preferably with conventional equipment).

Provided the above criteria are met, potential benefits derived from properly formulated controlled-release systems include: (1) enhanced agricultural production, (2) fewer applications, (3) less environmental pollution and (4) reduced production costs to the farmer.

Macromolecular Design

Polymeric systems for controlled-release of pesticides may be assigned to two broad categories. In the first, the pesticide is physically dissolved, entrapped, or dispersed in a polymer matrix. Chemical release is generally based on diffusion phenomena (14-19, 34-39); however, chemical or biological erosion of the polymer matrix is also possible. In the second category, the pesticide is chemically bound (pendant) to the macromolecular backbone. Release is then dependent on the rate of chemical or biological break-down of the polymer-to-pesticide bonds (20-24, 31-39).

Polymers containing pendant pesticides can be prepared by two synthetic methods. The first involves bonding (via covalent or ionic chemical bonds) of a pesticide to a pre-formed polymer. This approach requires macromolecules with pendant functional groups capable of reaction with pesticides or their derivatives. The nature of the chemical bond may be varied to yield bonds with quite different rates of cleavage in the environment. Advantages of this method include: (a) availability of relatively inexpensive polymers with biodegradability such as chitin, cellulose, etc., and (b) use of commercially available pesticides as starting materials in polymer synthesis.

The second approach involves polymerization of monomeric pesticides. The major advantages of this method lie in the ability to control the molecular design of the polymer and the pesticide/polymer weight ratio.

Experimental

Preformed, hydroxy-containing polymers were selected for initial study. Three polymers - polyvinyl alcohol, chitin, and cellulose were chose on the basis of: (a) potential biodegradability, (b) commercial availability, and (c) hydrophilicity in addition to having proper pendant functionality. The results of the experiments on polyvinyl alcohol are reported in this work.

Metribuzin was chosen as a model pesticide based on: (a) available amine functionality, (b) high activity at relatively low concentrations, (c) selectivity, (d) lack of persistence in the environment, and (e) high mobility.

A series of laboratory and commercial polymers of polyvinyl alcohol (with varying residual amounts of unhydrolyzed vinyl acetate) were carefully characterized. Isocyanate adducts of metribuzin were prepared and reacted with the pendant hydroxyl functionality of the pre-formed polymers (Figure 1). It was possible to prepare copolymers with varying degrees of substitution on linear and highly cross-linked chains.

The isocyanate to hydroxyl ratios were varied over a wide range to prepare solvent swollen, cross-linked gels. These were converted to microporous solids by agitation of the product in the presence of a non-solvent (selected from solubility parameter data).

Rates of Release of Metribuzin

Polymers with pendant metribuzin (0.100 g) were placed in an Erlenmeyer flask. 500 ml of distilled water was added. At designated intervals, samples were taken to determine the concentration of released metribuzin.

Ultraviolet Spectroscopic Method. A Cary 1756 Spectrophotometer was used to determine released metribuzin levels in water. A standard plot of absorbance vs. concentration was obtained using least squares analysis. 3 ml samples were taken at designated intervals and placed in standard quartz cells. The absorbance at 293.5 nm was monitored in two types of tests. The first measured total concentration of released metribuzin over a time period. The second test was conducted as follows: (a) 0.100 g samples were placed in 500 ml of distilled water for a predetermined time; (b) the samples were filtered, dried and again placed in a second Erlenmeyer flask containing 500 ml of distilled water; (c) concentrations were measured directly from the filtrate.

Gas Chromatographic Method. 2μl of aqueous solution were removed and extracted with 5.0 ml of benzene. 1 μl of the benzene phase was then injected into the gas chromatograph (Micro-Tek 220 with electron capture detector).

Soil Mobility Studies

Thin-layer plates were prepared by spreading a soil slurry onto 20 X 20 cm glass plates to a thickness of 1.0 mm. Plates were divided into three equal sections by scribing the soil layer. Metribuzin was applied to one plate by streaking 500 λ of a 100 g/ml solution onto each section of the plate 2 cm from the bottom. Polymers containing pendant metribuzin were embedded in

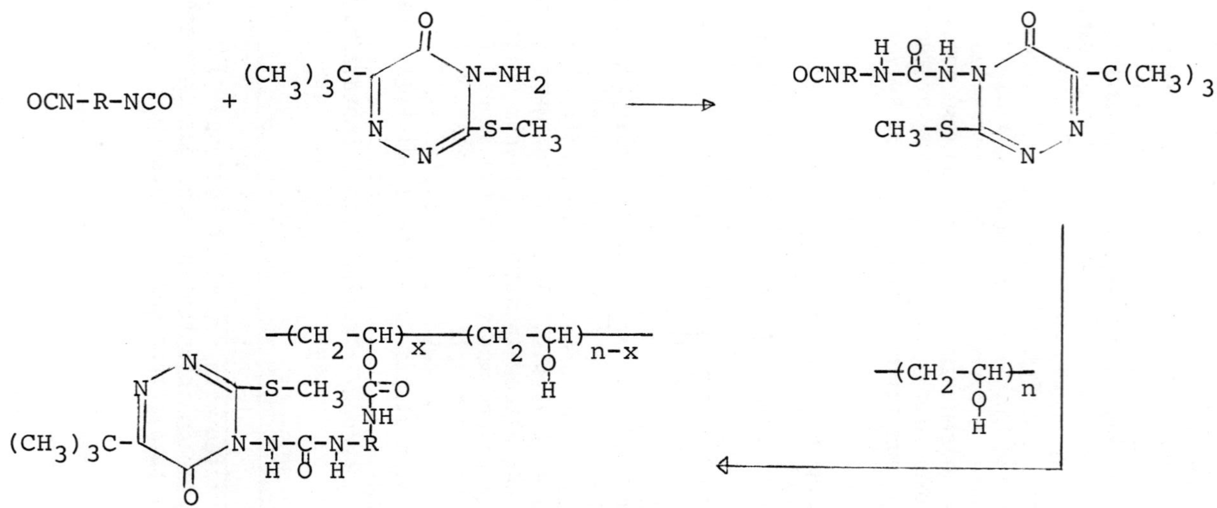

Figure 1. Synthetic method for preparation of PVA copolymer containing pendant metribuzin

the soil layer on other plates which were also divided into three sections. The plates were eluted to 10 cm with water, air dried, and 1-cm zones were removed from one of the three sections of each plate. The plates were returned to the chamber and again eluted with 10 cm of water, and the second zone was removed in 1-cm sections. This procedure was repeated with the third section of soil. The soil removed in this manner was extracted with 5 ml of hexane: acetone (3:1) by shaking. Extract was analyzed by gas chromatography.

Residual Phytotoxicity Of Metribuzin From Polymers

The polymers containing pendant metribuzin were added to the surface of a Bosket sandy loam soil contained in 4" plastic pots in a controlled-environment chamber. The application rates were 0, 0.1, 0.2, and 0.3 g of each formulation. A commercial formulation of metribuzin was applied to other pots at 0.5 and 1.0 ppmw, and thoroughly mixed into the soil. The soils were bioassayed over a period of 112 days with a mixture of weeds which are normally susceptible to the herbicide; after growing two weeks, the weeds were harvested and first weights recorded.

Results And Discussion

Five polymers containing pendant metribuzin were chosen for study: 22-S, 23-S, 41-S, 45-S, and 50-S. 23-S, 45-S, and 50-S were essentially linear polymers prepared from 99% hydrolyzed polyvinyl alcohol. 22-S and 41-S were highly cross-linked microporous solids. These system require both hydrolysis of the urea bond and diffusion from a water swollen, cross-linked matrix for metribuzin release.

Plots of solution concentration vs. time (Figures 2, 3) indicated that the linear polymers (23-S, 45-S, and 50-S) released herbicide much more rapidly than the cross-linked systems. The 23-S, 45-S, and 50-S were characterized by a rapid initial release in the first few hours followed by a more gradual rate lasting several days. The cross-linked systems 22-S and 41-S (Figure 4) had much lower release rates with little initial release. This could be predicted by the time required for swelling of the hydrophilic polymer so that hydrolysis and diffusion could occur. After swelling, slight concentration increases were noted. The u.v. spectroscopic data and the gas chromatographic data were internally consistent. It should be noted that the ultraviolet technique requires no extraction and, therefore, offers less chance for error at small concentrations of metribuzin.

Soil thin-layer chromatographic techniques showed metribuzin (Figure 5) moved as a normal chromatogram peak with each successive elution moving the peak nearer the 10-cm zone. The chromatograms from 23-S (Figure 6) and 45-S (Figure 7) showed "streaking" continuously along the plate indicating a sustained release mechanism. The cross-linked formulations, 22-S and 45-S,

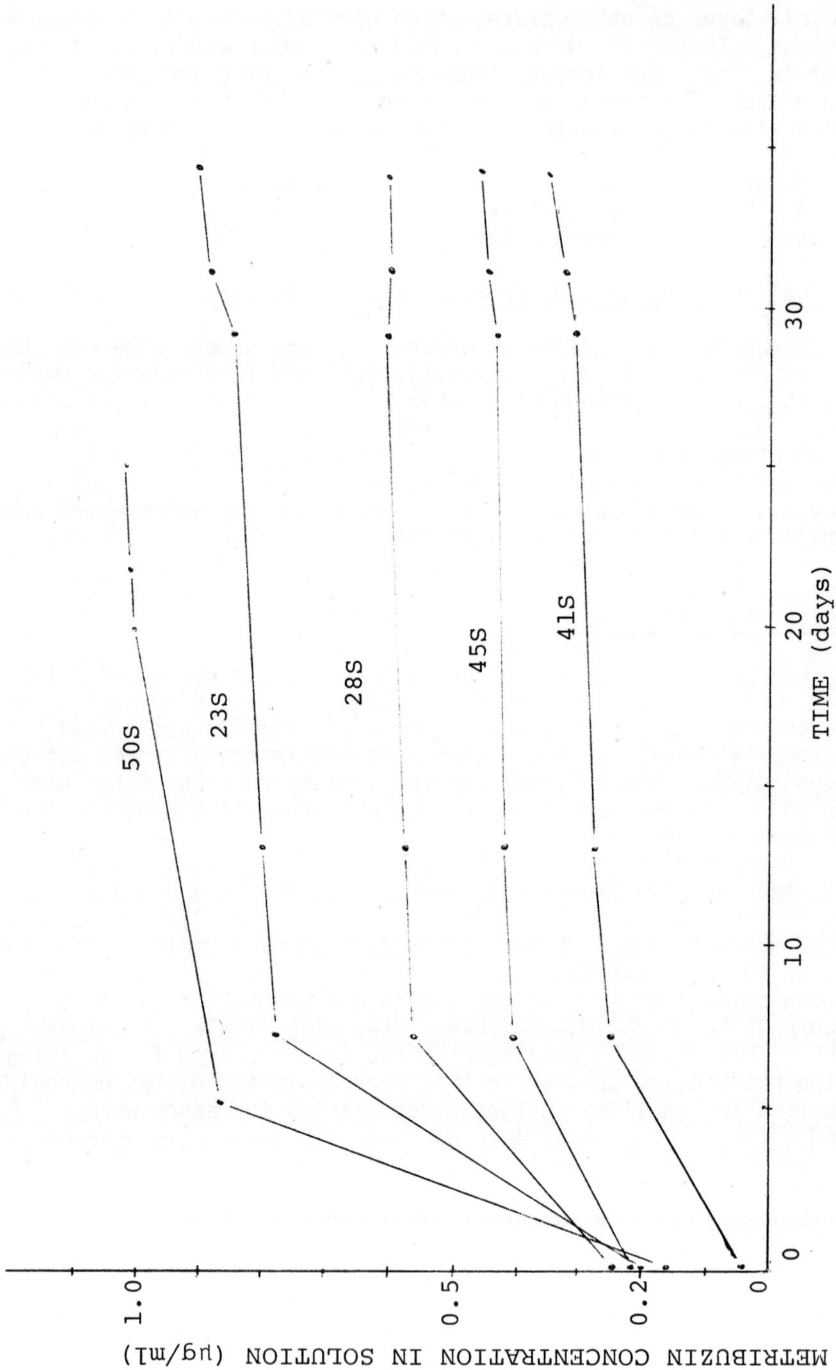

Figure 2. Metribuzin release from polymers in water (ultraviolet spectroscopy)

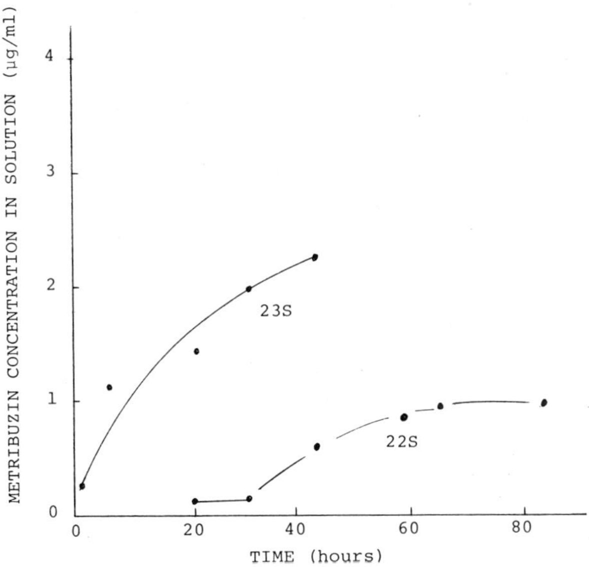

Figure 3. Metribuzin release from linear (23S) and cross-linked (22S) polymers

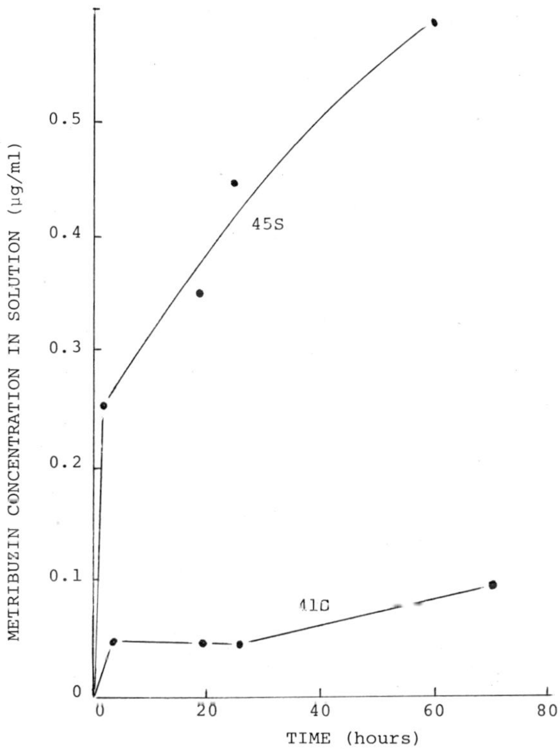

Figure 4. Metribuzin release from linear (45S) and cross-linked (41S) polymers

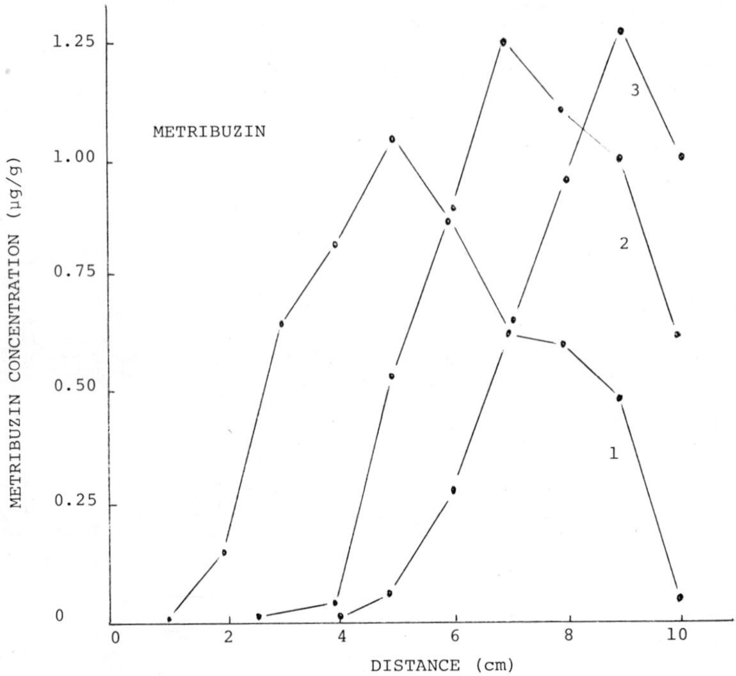

Figure 5. Soil thin layer chromatography (TLC) of metribuzin

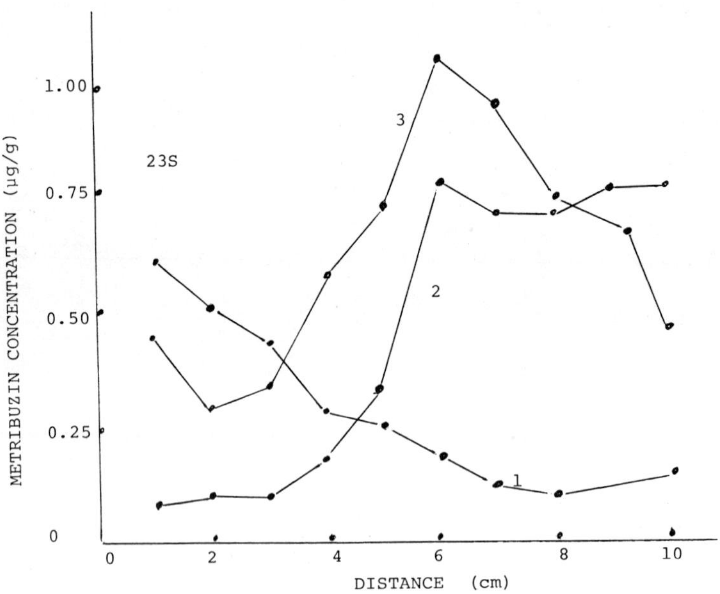

Figure 6. Soil TLC of metribuzin released from 23S

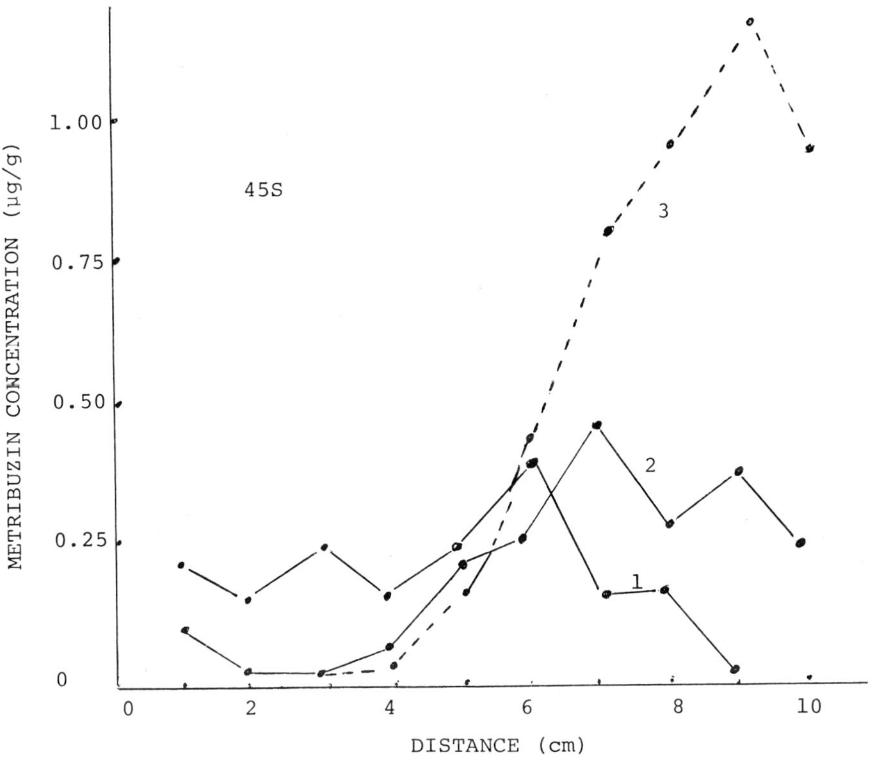

Figure 7. Soil TLC of metribuzin released from 45S

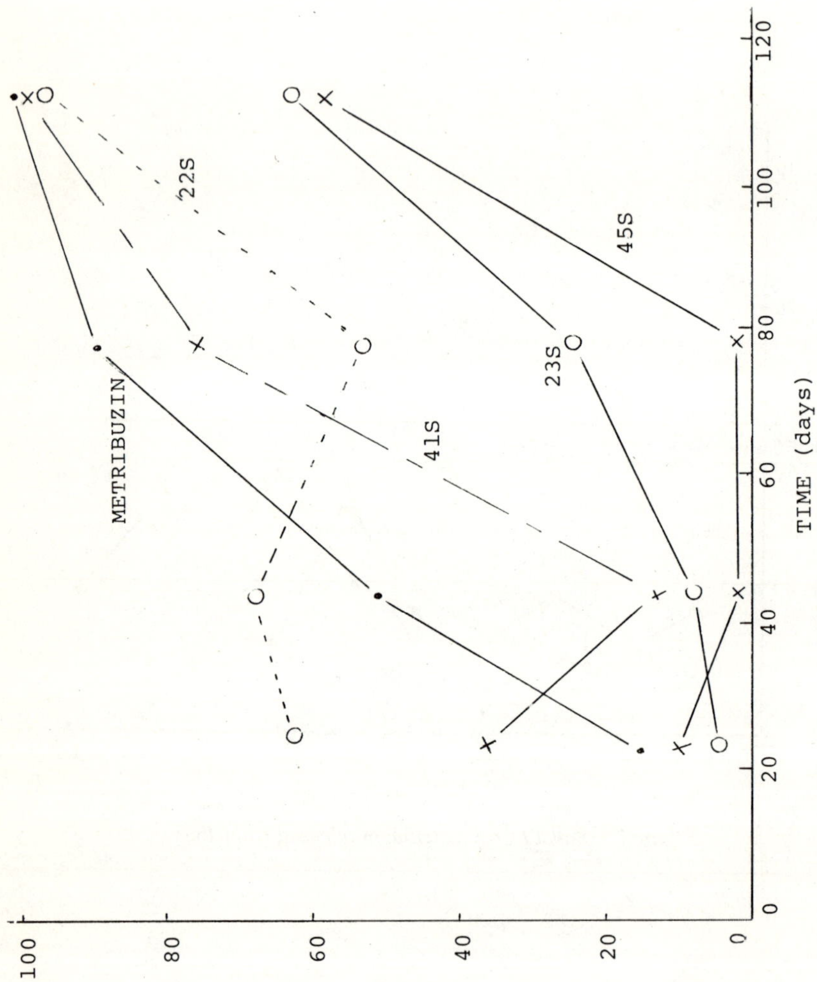

Figure 8. Phytotoxicity of metribuzin from polymer formulations as a function of time

did not release enough metribuzin for a measurable rate in these studies.

Residual phytotoxicity of the four polymeric systems is illustrated in Figure 8. Metribuzin at 1.0 ppmw had dissipated to a level which was essentially non-toxic after 78 days. Likewise, phytotoxicity from 41-S had diminished to a large extent by this time. A relatively low level of phytoxicity was observed for 22-S initially; however, this same level was maintained for over 78 days, then rapidly decreased.

The highest level of phytotoxicity was observed with 23-S and 45-S. These materials were still showing phytotoxicity at our last test date of 112 days.

It must be noted that phytotoxicity comparison tests of polymeric controlled-release formulations and commercially formulated herbicides must be interpreted with care. In the pendant polymeric systems, herbicides are not phytotoxic until bond cleavage has occurred. For this reason the total herbicide eventually available in the polymer cannot be compared to that immediately available in a commercial formulation.

Conclusions

Polymeric systems for controlled release of metribuzin have been prepared using biodegradable substrates. Properly selected macromolecular substrates were reacted with pesticide adducts to yield systems with labile pesticide-to-polymer bonds susceptible to chemical or enzymatic hydrolysis.

The metribuzin/polyvinyl alcohol system in this work is adaptable for formation of a range of products with different degrees of cross-linking and, therefore, different rates of herbicide release. Phytotoxicity, soil thin-layer chromatography, ultraviolet spectroscopy, and gas chromatography tests showed sustained release capabilities of the polymeric systems.

The preliminary results of this research point to the immense potential of polymeric systems for controlled-release of selective herbicides which can: (1) reduce environmental pollution in non-target areas by reducing pesticide mobility, (2) require fewer applications during the growing season, and (3) result in enhanced agricultural production at, perhaps, lower cost to the farmer.

Acknowledgements

The authors would like to express their thanks for the generous support of research conducted at the University of Southern Mississippi Polymer Science Laboratories provided by Hopkins Agricultural Chemical Company of Madison, Wisconsin. Research support was also obtained from the USDA Weed Science Laboratories at Stoneville, Mississippi, and from the Mississippi-Alabama Sea Grant Program. The soil studies were conducted by

K. E. Savage, Southern Weed Science Lab., ARS, USDA, Stoneville, MS, 38776.

Abstract

Recently, there has been a growing interest in developing pesticide controlled release technology. Much of the impetus has resulted from demands for enhanced agricultural production at lower levels of environmental risk. Most of the activity has been directed toward formulations in which the pesticide is physically dissolved or dispersed in a polymer matrix. Polymers have been prepared in our laboratories which contain labile polymer to pesticide covalent bonds. These linkages are susceptible to aqueous and/or bacterial break-down, resulting in long-term release. Theoretically, the rate of herbicide release can be controlled by changing the nature of the labile bonds or by altering the cross-link density of the polymer. The synthesized systems have been characterized by IR, NMR, U.V., GPC, etc. Release studies have been conducted in aqueous media using U.V. and gas chromatography. In addition, soil mobility and phytotoxicity studies are in progress.

Literature Cited

1. Barrett, B. B., Louisiana Wildlife and Fisheries Commission Report, Cooperative Gulf of Mexico Estuarine Inventory and Study, Hydrology, p. 115, 1971.
2. Christmas, J.Y., Ed., Cooperative Gulf of Mexico Estuarine Inventory and Study, Mississippi, Publishers: Gulf Coast Research Laboratory, p. 12, 1973.
3. Chemical and Engineering News, July 28, 1975, pp. 18-31.
4. Kearney, R.C. and Kaufman, D.D., Herbicides, Chemistry, Degradation, and Mode of Action, 2nd Edition, Marcel Dekker, Inc., 1975.
5. Butler, P.A., Pesticide Monitoring Journal, Vol. 6(4) 238, 1973.
6. Butler, P.A., "Pesticides in the Estuary," Proc. of Marsh and Estuary Management Symposium (July 1967), Baton Rouge, LA, pp. 120-124, 1968.
7. Butler, P.A., Proc. of National Symposium on Estuarine Pollution, (August, 1967) Stanford University, p. 107, 1968.
8. Butler, P.A., "Significance of DDT Residue in Estuarine Fauna," Chemical Fallout, Chapter 9, pp. 205-220, 1969.
9. "Pesticides in the Marine Environment," Journal Appl. Ecology 3, (Supplement) pp. 253-259, 1966.
10. "Problems of Pesticides in Estuaries," American Fish Soc., SPE Public No. 3, pp. 110-115, 1966.
11. Firth, F.E., Ed., "Pesticides in the Sea," Encyclopedia of Marine Resources, pp. 513-516.
12. Butler, P.A., "Pesticides," U.S. Bureau of Commercial Fisheries Report: Contract No. 85, 1967.

13. Andus, L.J., Ed., The Physiology and Biochemistry of Herbicides, Academic Press, New York, 1964.
14. U.S. Patent #3,074,845.
15. U.S. Patent #3,318,769.
16. U.S. Patent #3,737,521.
17. U.S. Patent #3,127,752.
18. U.S. Patent #3,400,093.
19. U.S. Patent #3,343,941.
20. Allan, G.C., et al. Nature, 234, 349 (1971).
21. Neogi, A.N., Ph.D., Thesis University of Washington, Seattle, Washington, (1970).
22. Jakube, H.D., Busch, E., F. Chem, 13 (3), p. 105 (1973).
23. Allan, G.C., et al. Int. Pest Control, 14 (2), p. 15 (1972).
24. Harris, F.W. and Post, L.K., Polymer Preprints, 16 (1), pp. 622-627, (1975).
25. Pariser, E.R. and Block, S., Chitin and Chitin Derivatives, Report No. MITSG 73-2, October 15, 1972, (A bibliography with 593 references).
26. Davidson, R.L. and Sittig, Marshall, Eds., Water-Soluble Resins, Van Nonstrand Reinhold Co., New York, 1968.
27. Bikales, N.M., Water-Soluble Polymers, Plenum Press, New York, 1973.
28. O'Brien, R.D., Insecticides, Action and Metabolism, Academic Press, New York, 1967.
29. White-Stevens, R., Pesticides in the Environment, Marcel Dekker, 1973.
30. Chemical Engineering, January 19, 1976.
31. Allan, G.C., Canadian Patent #846785.
32. Allan, G.C., Canadian Patent #863310.
33. Allan, G.C., Canadian Patent #855181.
34. Chemical and Engineering News, June 28, 1976.
35. Controlled Release Pesticide Symposium, The University of Akron, September, 1974.
36. Proceedings 1975 International Controlled Release Pesticide Symposium, Wright State University, September, 1975.
37. Proceedings 1976 Controlled Release Pesticide Symposium, The University of Akron, September, 1976.
38. Cardarelli, N., Controlled Release Pesticides Formulations, CRC Press, Cleveland, Ohio, 1976.
39. Paul, D.R. and Harris, F.W., Eds., Controlled Release Polymeric Formulations, ACS Symposium Series, 33, 1976.

12

Microencapsulated Pesticides

HERBERT B. SCHER

Formulations Section, Chemical Research Department, Stauffer Chemical Co., 1200 So. 47th St., Richmond, Calif. 94804

Microcapsules are 1-200 micron particles composed of a solid or liquid core surrounded by a wall. The wall is generally polymeric in nature (Figure 1) and constitutes 5-25 percent of the microcapsule by weight. The wall isolates and protects the core material in storage but is designed to release the core material in a controlled fashion when the microcapsules are exposed to the environment. The core material can be released from the microcapsules by crushing the wall, breaking the wall by pressure from within, dissolving the wall, hydrolyzing the wall or by diffusing through the wall.

Controlled release of pesticides (insecticides, herbicides, fungicides, fumigants, juvenile hormone mimics, insect sex attractants and animal health compounds) can be achieved by microencapsulation. Pesticide microcapsule systems can be designed to:

1. Reduce mammalian toxicity and extend activity.
2. Reduce evaporative losses.
3. Reduce phytotoxicity.
4. Protect pesticides from environmental degradation.
5. Reduce leaching.
6. Reduce pesticide levels in the environment.

An aqueous dispersion of pesticide microcapsules is a particularly useful controlled release pesticide formulation because:

1. It is composed of discrete microcapsules as opposed to aggregates.
2. It can be diluted with water or liquid fertilizers and sprayed using conventional equipment. Uniform field coverage of pesticide is possible.
3. It requires less polymeric component per pound of pesticide than monolithic devices.
4. It is capable of establishing a constant pesticide release rate (See Figures 2 and 3).

Gelatin	Polyethers
Gum Arabic	Polyesters
Starch	Polyamides
Sugar	Polyureas
Ethyl Cellulose	Polybutadiene
Carboxymethyl Cellulose	Polyisoprene
Paraffin	Polysiloxanes
Polyvinyl alcohol	Polyurethanes
Polyethylene	Epoxy resins
Polypropylene	inorganic silicates
Polystyrene	
Polyacrylamide	

Encyclopedia of Polymer Science and Technology

Figure 1. Common microcapsule wall materials

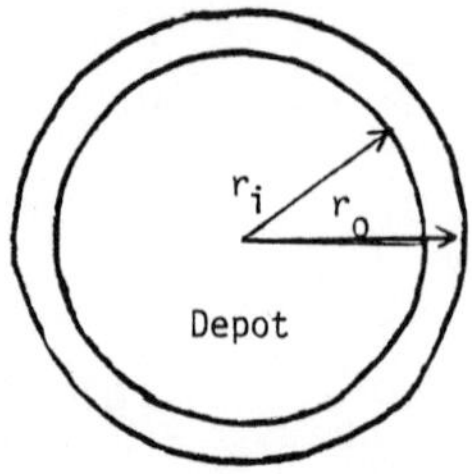

$$\frac{dM}{dt} = \text{Release Rate} = 4\pi DK \, \Delta C \, \frac{r_o r_i}{r_o - r_i}$$

D = Diffusion Coefficient

K = Distribution Coefficient

DK = Permeability

Δ C = Concentration Difference Across Wall

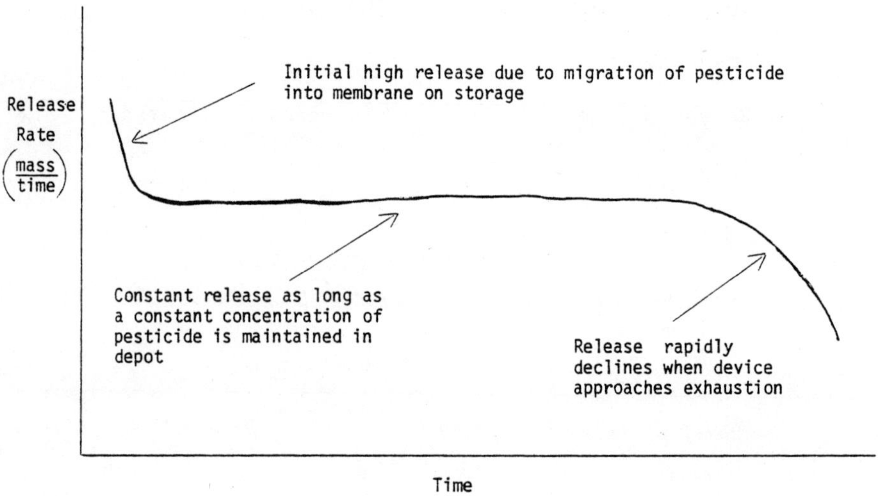

Chemical Technology

Figure 2. Pesticide release rate from microcapsule (2)

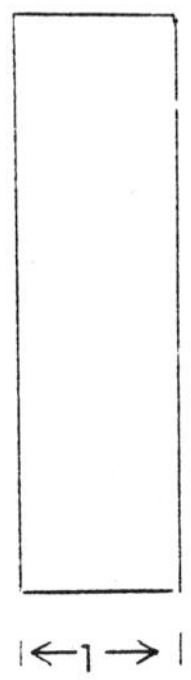

(SLAB GEOMETRY)

Dissolved Pesticide

$$\frac{dM}{dt} = 2M_\infty \left(\frac{D}{\pi l^2 t}\right)^{1/2} \quad \text{for } 0 \leq \frac{M}{M_\infty} \leq 0.6$$

$$\frac{dM}{dt} = \frac{8DM_\infty}{2} \exp\left(\frac{-\pi^2 Dt}{l^2}\right) \quad \text{for } 0.4 \leq \frac{M}{M_\infty} \leq 1.0$$

where D = Diffusion coefficient

t = time

M_∞ = Total mass of pesticide

Dispersed Pesticide

$$\frac{dM}{dt} = M_\infty \left(\frac{2DC_s}{C_o l^2 t}\right)^{1/2}$$

C_o = total concentration of agent in matrix

C_s = solubility of agent in matrix

$\frac{dM}{dt}$ = release rate

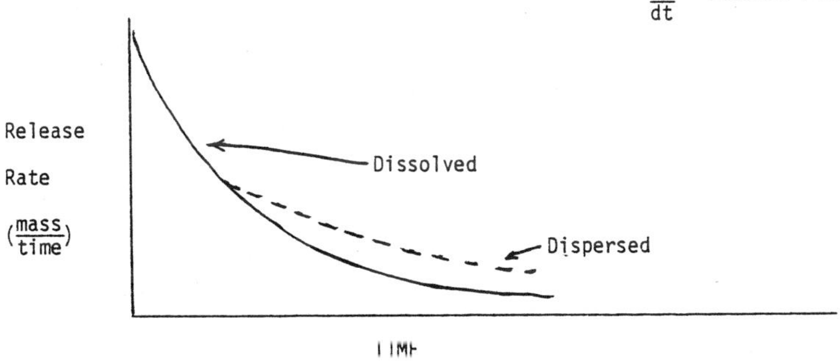

Chemical Technology

Figure 3. Pesticide release rate from monolithic device (2)

5. The pesticide release rate can be varied over wide limits by varying the microcapsule particle size distribution, the microcapsule wall thickness and the microcapsule wall permeability. Mixtures of different microcapsules can also be used to adjust the pesticide release rate.
6. Additives such as film forming agents can be added directly to the formulation. These agents can improve the adhesion of microcapsules to foliage.

Microencapsulation processes can be divided into three categories (3)(4). In the Phase Separation category, microcapsules are formed by emulsifying or dispersing the core material in an immiscible continuous phase in which the wall material is dissolved and then the wall material is caused to physically seperate from the continuous phase and deposit around the core particles. In the Interfacial Reaction category, microcapsules are formed by emulsifying or dispersing the core material in an immiscible continuous phase and then an interfacial polymerization reaction is caused to take place at the surface of the core particles. In the Physical Methods category, wall material and core particles are physically brought together and the wall flows around the core particle to form the microcapsule.

Microencapsulation processes are listed below according to these three categories.

I. Phase Separation Methods

a. Aqueous Phase Separation (complex coacervation) - National Cash Register Company.
b. Organic Phase Separation - I.B.M.
c. Meltable Disperion - National Cash Register Company.
d. Spray Drying - Moore Business Forms, National Starch and Chemical Corporation.
e. Fluidized-Bed Spray Coating - Smith, Kline and French; Wisconsin Alumini Research Foundation.

II. Interfacial Reactions

a. Interfacial Condensation Polymerization - Pennwalt Chemical Company.
b. In Situ Interfacial Condensation Polymerization - Stauffer Chemical Company
c. Interfacial Addition Polymerization - Stanford Research Institute; National Cash Register Company.

III. Physical Methods

a. Multiorifice Centrifugal - Southwest Research Institute.
b. Electrostatic - IIT Research Institute.

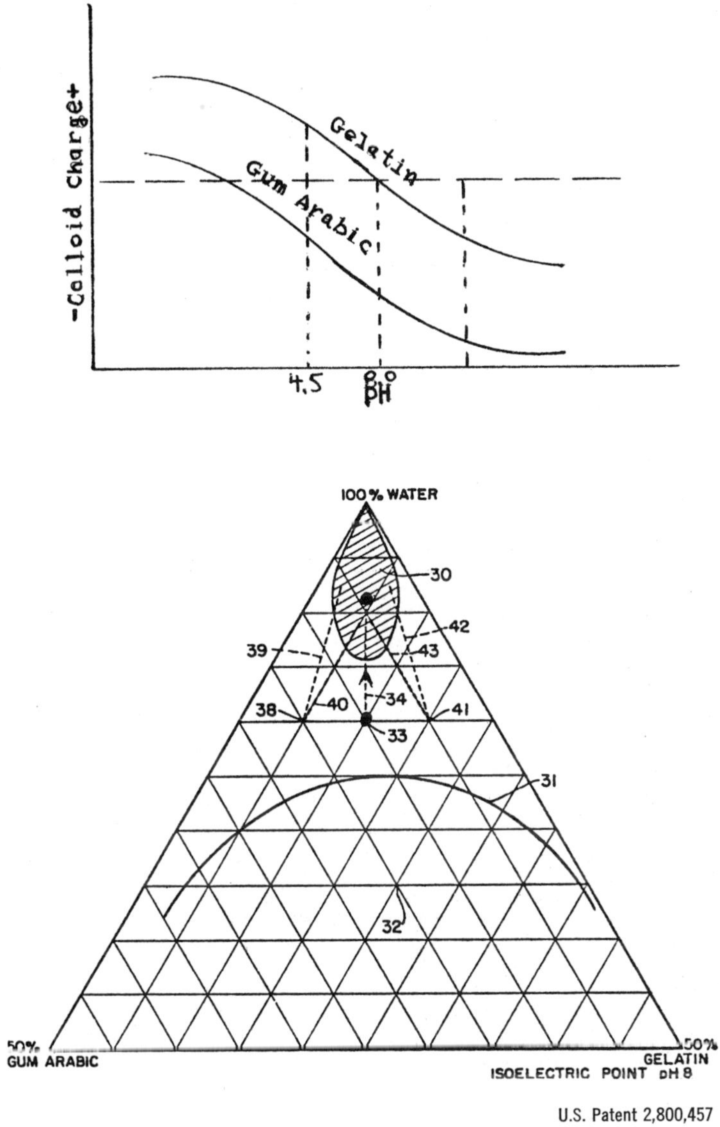

Figure 4. Complex coacervation

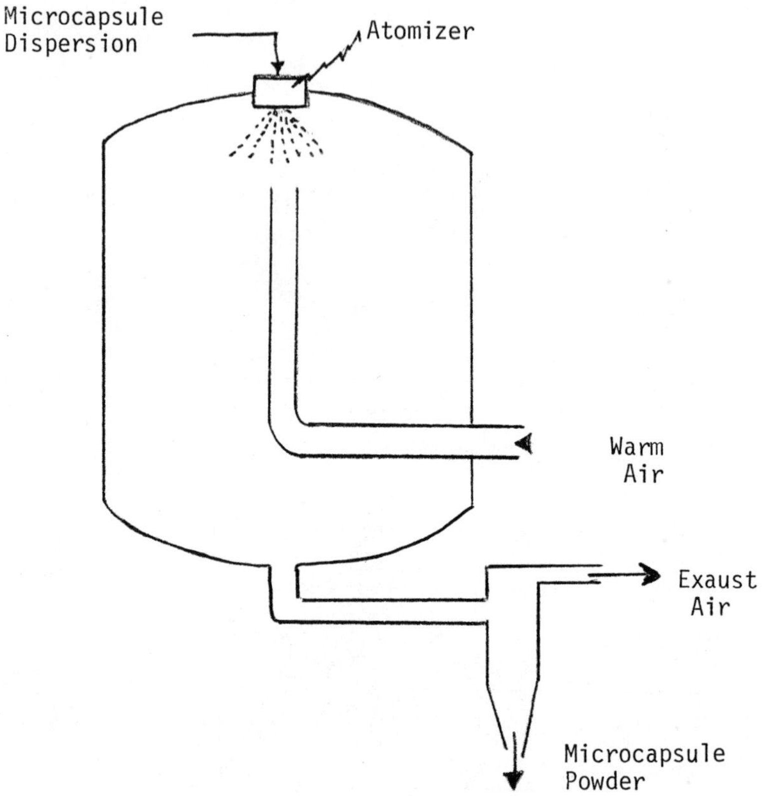

Encyclopedia of Polymer Science and Technology

Figure 5. Spray dryers are direct, dispersion-type dryers which operate on the principle of atomizing a fluid feed to form a spray of droplets which mix with hot gases to evaporate a liquid and produce a dispersed, dry product. Spray dryers find extensive application in the process and food industries. They can be characterized as follows: (1) an atomizing device disperses the liquid into a spray of droplets with a range of drop sizes. Drops can range in diameter from 100–600 μ depending on the type of atomizer used, the capacity, and atomizing conditions. (2) Hot gases, introduced by a variety of gas-inlet configurations, contact the spray and evaporate moisture from the individual drops. (3)The mixture of hot gases and spray droplets which produce a dry, particulate product has a residence time in the dryer which is highly statistical in character. (4) The dry product and drying gases must be separated to obtain the desired dry product in the form of finely divided material. (5) Any residual product must be recovered from the exhaust gases.

Aqueous Phase Separation (complex coacervation), Interfacial Condensation Polymerization and In Situ Interfacial Condensation Polymerization are the most widely used processes for microencapsulating pesticides. The resulting product of all three of these processes is an aqueous dispersion of pesticide microcapsules.

The National Cash Register Company (5) has used an aqueous phase separation process (complex coacervation) to microencapsulate pesticides for 20-years. The complex coacervation process consists of the following steps.

1. Dissolve gelatin (isoelectric point = 8) in aqueous phase (pH > 8.0; 50°C).
2. Emulsify pesticide liquid in aqueous phase.
3. Add gum arabic solution to aqueous phase (pH > 8.0; 50°C)
4. Mutual precipitation (complex coacervation) of gum arabic and gelatin around pesticide particles is induced by dropping pH to 4.5 and diluting with water (see Figure 4).
5. Gel complex coacervate by cooling to 5-10°C.
6. Harden complex coacervate by addition of glutaraldehyde or formaldehyde and adjusting pH to 9-10.

Organic Phase Separation (6) and Meltable Dispersion (7) processes are the inverse of Aqueous Phase Separation and are used to microencapsulate hydrophilic substances. Organic phase soluble polymers are precipitated around the hydrophilic core by the addition of a nonsolvent or cooling. Since pesticides are primarily lipophilic substances, these processes are generally not suitable for the microencapsulation of pesticides.

Spray Drying (8) and Fluidized Bed Spray Coating (9) are useful processes for the microencapsulation of pesticide solid particles. In the spray drying process, a film forming polymer is dissolved in the aqueous continuous phase of a pesticide dispersion. The drying process (see Figure 5) causes the water to evaporate and the polymer coats the pesticide particle. The resulting microcapsule product is a free-flowing, dry powder. In the Wurster process (Fluidized-Bed Spray Coating), a fluidized bed of solid pesticide particles is sprayed with an aqueous polymer solution. Coating of the pesticide particles occurs when the water is evaporated. Additional coats of polymer can be applied to the pesticide particles by recirculation through the spraying and drying zones (see Figure 6).

Pennwalt Corporation has pioneered in microencapsulation by interfacial condensation polymerization (10). Pencap M (microencapsulated Methyl Parathion) is produced by the interfacial reaction of sebacoyl chloride (in the organic phase) and ethylenediamine and diethylenetriamine (in the aqueous phase). The reaction product (microcapsule wall) is a cross linked polyamide (see Figure 7).

Stauffer Chemical Company has developed a microencapsulation process based on in situ interfacial condensation polymerization (11). The process is capable of producing an aqueous dispersion

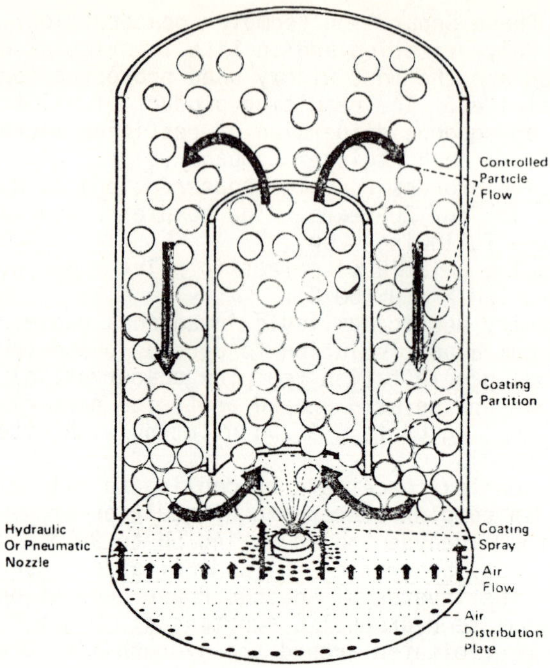

Microencapsulation Processes and Applications

Figure 6. Fluidized bed spray coating

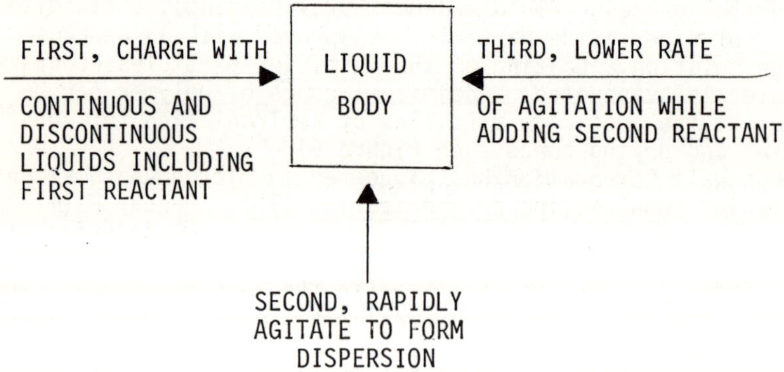

U.S. Patent 3,577,515

Figure 7. Interfacial condensation polymerization (10)

of microcapsules containing 4-pounds of active ingredient per gallon.

The first step of the process consists of dispersing an organic pesticide phase (containing isocyanate monomers) into a aqueous phase. The isocyanate monomers used in the process are polymethylene polyphenyl isocyanate (PAPI) and toluene diisocyanate (TDI). The wall forming reaction is initiated by heating the batch to an elevated temperature at which point the isocyanate monomers are hydrolyzed at the interface to form amines, which in turn react with unhydrolyzed isocyanate monomers to form the polyurea microcapsule wall. The process and wall forming reaction is described in Figure 8.

The release rate of this microcapsule system can be varied by varying microcapsule particle size (i.e., total surface area per pound of pesticide), wall thickness (weight percent isocyanate monomers in organic phase), and wall permeability. The wall permeability can be varied by varying the cross link density of the polyurea (ratio of PAPI to TDI). Electron scanning photomicrographs of the microcapsules produced by this process are shown in Figures 9-11.

Microencapsulation by interfacial addition polymerization (12) involves 1) dissolving vinyl monomers in pesticide liquid, 2) emulsifying pesticide solution in aqueous phase, 3) contacting surface of pesticide particle with addition polymerization catalyst.

Pesticide microcapsule powders can be produced by (13) multiorifice centrifugation (see Figure 12) or (14) electrostatic encapsulation (see Figure 13). The diameters of the microcapsules produced by these physical methods are limited to 80 μ and larger.

The factors affecting the rate of release of the core material from a microcapsule were smmarized by (15) Fanger (see Figure 14).

The following examples show the variety of applications for microencapsulated pesticides.

1. Microencapsulated Methyl Parathion (Pencap M produced by Pennwalt Corp.)
   Microencapsulating Methyl Parathion reduces its mammalian toxicity and extends its activity (16)
2. Microencapsulated juvenile hormone (Altosid produced by Zoecon)
   Microencapsulation protects this juvenile hormone from environmental degradation (17)
3. Microencapsulated Disparlure (gypsy moth sex attractant)
   Microencapsulation controls the evaporation of Disparlure and extends its activity (18)
4. Microencapsulated Mirex
   Microcapsules of 2% Mirex in vegetable oil are very attractive to the imported fire ant and give a high degree of control. The ability of microencapsulated

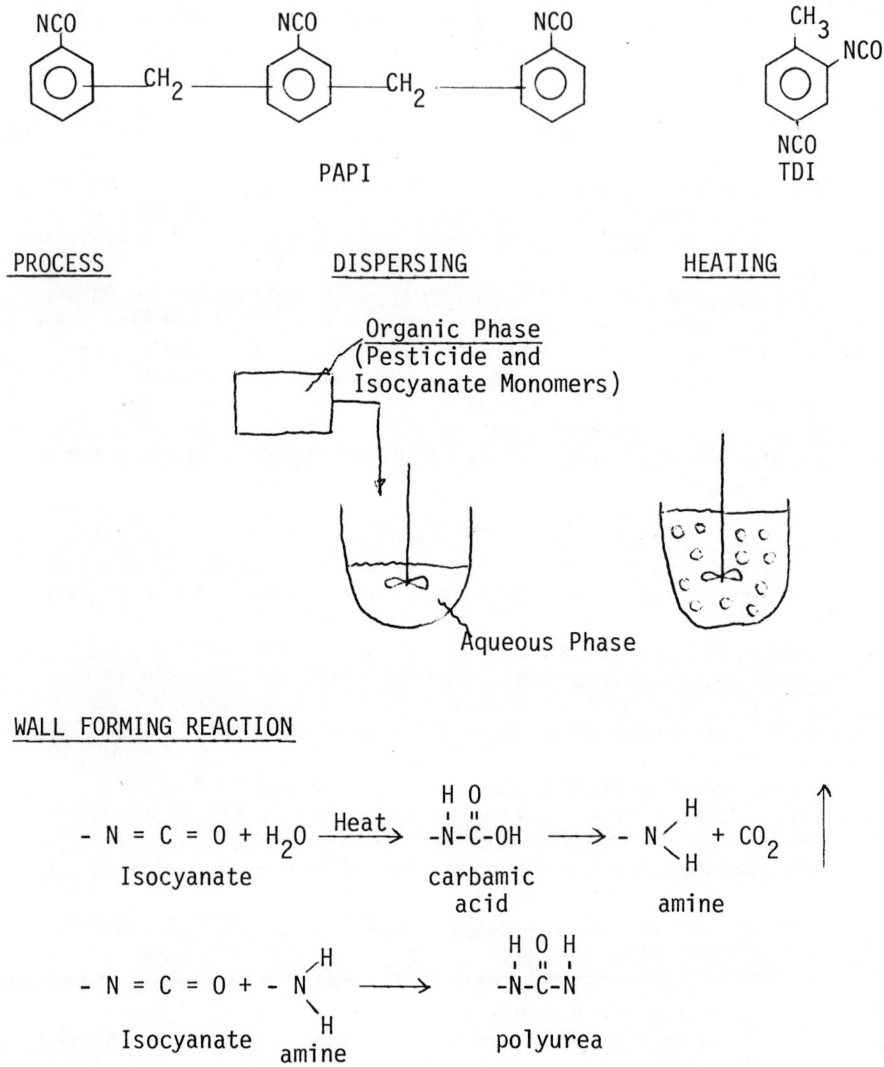

Great Britain Patent 1,371,179

Figure 8. In situ interfacial condensation polymerization (11)

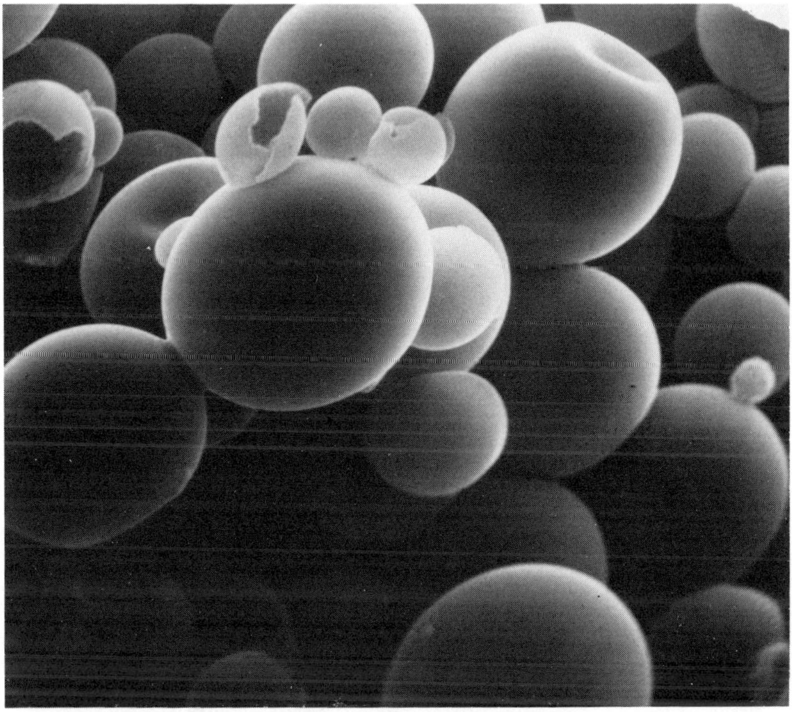

Figure 9. Magnification: 1000×; particle size distribution = 10–40 μ. Note the smooth membrane-like outer wall surface and the crushed capsules in upper left corner revealing thin wall.

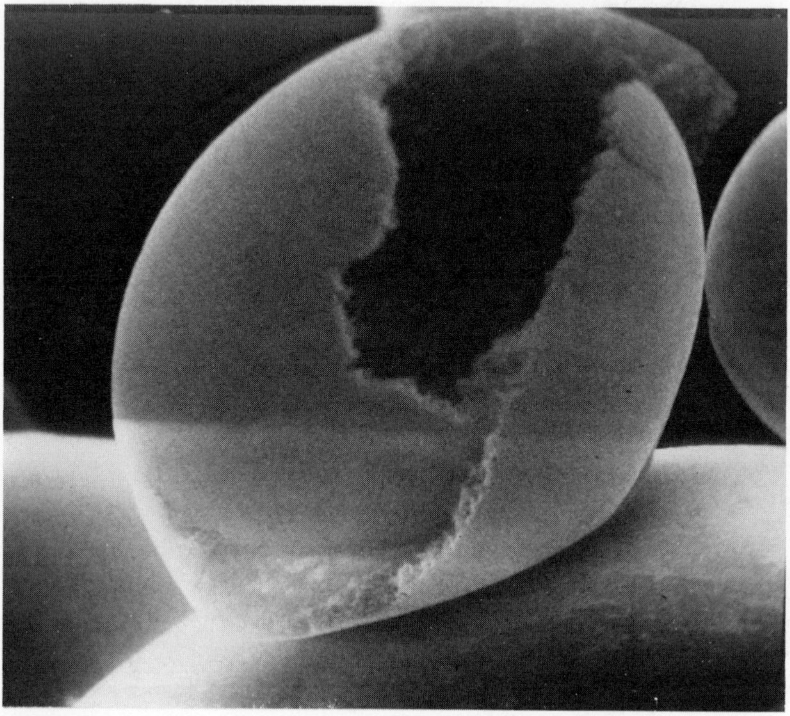

Figure 10. Magnification: 6000×. Note the smooth membrane-like outer wall surface and the sponge-like nature of the wall interior.

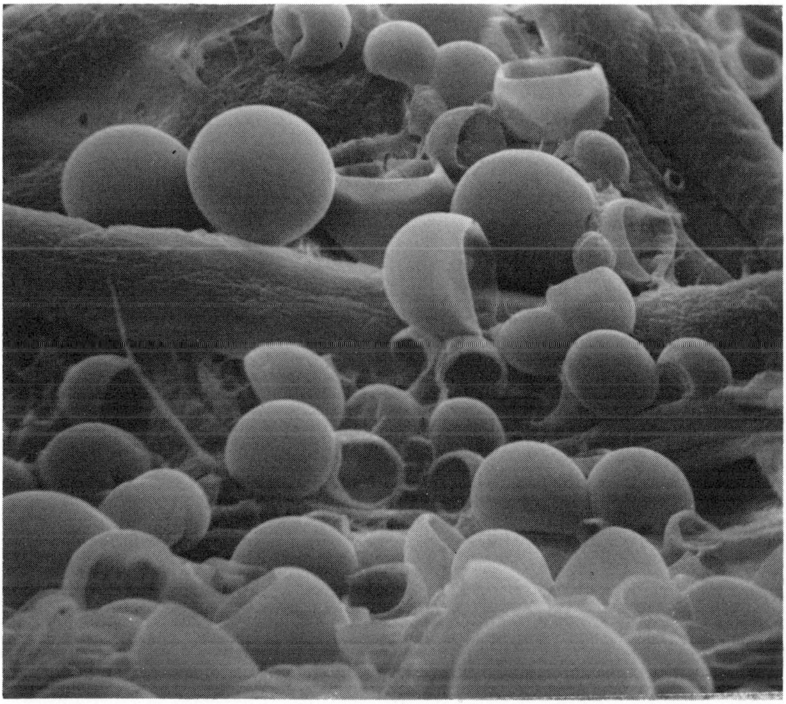

Figure 11. Microcapsules on cellulose filter. Magnification: 1000×. Note the cellulose fibers and the collapse of capsules as the pesticide diffuses through wall.

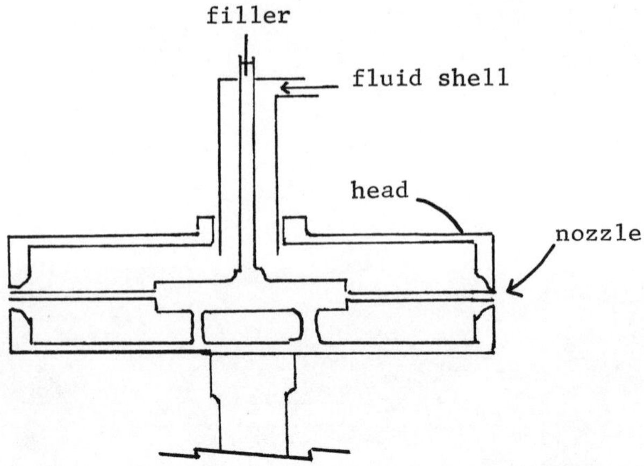

Chemical Engineering

Figure 12. Multiorifice centrifugation. The centrifugal extruder consists of a rotating head with nozzles on the periphery. Capsule filler, pumped into the inner chamber, flows through the tubes that project into orifices at the periphery of the head. Fluid-shell formulation, pumped into the head, flows through the anuli formed by the orifices and filler tubes. The result, in effect, is the extrusion of fluid "rods" of filler sheathed in fluid-shell formulations. These rods subsequently break into individual fluid capsules that are hardened by chemical reactions, evaporation, cooling, or other means.

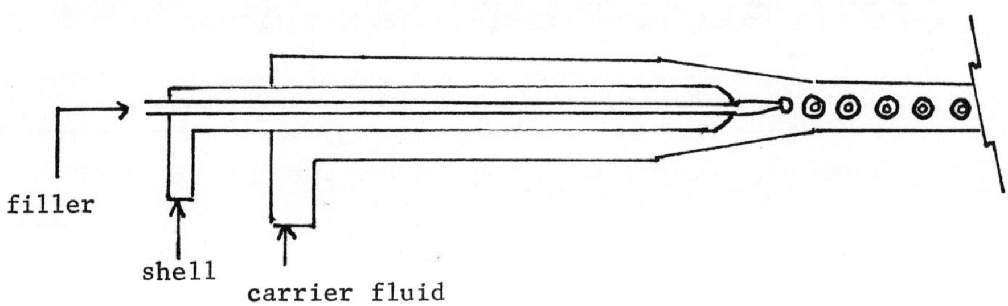

Chemical Engineering

Figure 12 (continued). *The extrusion nozzle device has two concentric tubes mounted axially in a tubular duct. Capsule filter is pumped through the center tube and fluid-shell formulation through the anulus of the nozzle so as to extrude a coated filler "rod" which breaks into individual capsules that are carried away in the stream of nonreactive carrier fluid. Capsule size is a function of the relative velocities of carrier fluid and extruded materials.*

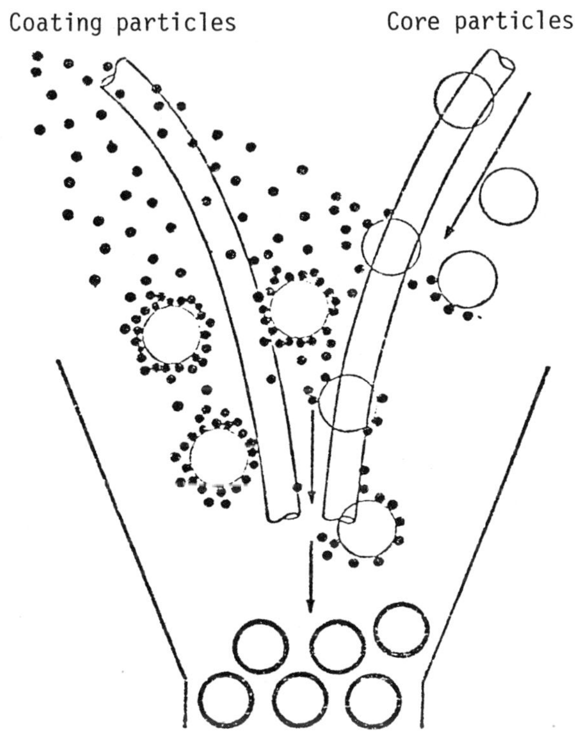

Chemical Engineering

Figure 13. The principle of electrostatic encapsulation. The two aerosols, produced separately in atomizers, bear opposite electric charges that greatly increase the attraction of core and coating particles. After coalescing, the coating droplets flow together to form a continuous film on the core. A subsequent cooling step then solidifies the coating, and capsules are gathered as a dry powder. Wet collection may also be used.

POLYMERIC WALL MATERIAL	FOR LOWER PERMEABILITY
PARAMETERS (1)	
Density	Increase
Crystallinity	Increase
Orientation	Increase
Crosslinking	Increase
Plasticizer Level	Decrease
Fillers	(Increase) Conditional
Solvents Used in Film Preparation	Use Good Solvents Versus Poor
Solubility Paramter (2)	One the Opposite Side of SP Scale From Core Material
CAPSULAR PARAMETERS	
Size	Increase
Wall Thickness	Increase
Configuration	As Spherical As Possible
Conformity	As Regular As Possible
Post Treatments (Crosslinking, Sintering)	Utilize
Multiple Coatings	Utilize
ENVIRONMENTAL PARAMETERS	
Temperature, Storage	Decrease
Partial Pressure Differential (Inside and Outside of Capsule Wall)	Decrease

Microencapsulation Processes and Applications

Figure 14. Parameters affecting capsular wall permeability

bait to withstand weathering makes it superior to corncob grits bait in controlling the ant during certain seasons. Aerial application of microencapsulated bait is feasible (19).

5. Microencapsulated Bacillus Thuringiensis (Bacterium)

The bacterium Bacillus thuringiensis, encapsulated by several processes, retained its viability and pathogenicity for the European corn borer. In field tests the capsule formulation was applied dry and in spray form, giving good control in both (20).

The uses and examples discussed above seem to indicate that pesticide microcapsule formulations have a bright future in agriculture.

Abstract

Controlled release of pesticides can be achieved by microencapsulation. Pesticide microcapsule systems can be designed to reduce mammalian toxicity and extend activity; reduce evaporative losses; reduce phytotoxicity; protect pesticides from environmental degradation; reduce leaching; reduce pesticide levels in the environment.

An aqueous dispersion of pesticide microcapsules is a particularly useful controlled release formulation because it is composed of discrete microcapsules; it can be diluted with water or liquid fertilizers and sprayed using conventional equipment; it requires less polymeric component per pound of pesticide than monolithic devices; it is capable of establishing a constant pesticide release rate; pesticide release rate can be varied over wide limits by varying microcapsule particle size distribution, wall thickness, and wall permeability; additives such as film forming agents can be added directly to the formulation.

Microencapsulation processes are grouped into three categories (Phase Separation, Interfacial Reactions and Physical Methods) and reviewed with respect to application to pesticides. Factors affecting the permeability of a pesticide through a microcapsule wall are also summarized.

Examples are given to show the variety of agricultural uses to which microencapsulated pesticides can be applied.

Literature Cited

(1) Baker, R. W. and Lonsdale, H. K., "Controlled Release of Biological Active Agents", Tanquary, A. C., and Lacey, R. E., editors, P. 15, Plenum Press, New York (1974).

(2) Baker, R. W. and Lonsdale, H. K., Chem. Tech. (1975), 5, 668-674.

(3) Flinn, J. E. and Nack, H., Chem. Eng. (1967), 74, 171-178.
(4) Wolfgang, S., Angew. Chem. Internat. Edit. (1975), 14, 539-550.
(5) Gutcho, M. H., "Microcapsules and Microencapsulation Techniques", P. 8, Noyes Data Corporation, Park Ridge, N.J., (1976).
(6) Reyes, Z., U.S. Patent 3,173,878 (1965).
(7) Herbig, J. A. and Hanny, J. F., U.S. Patent 3,161,602 (1964).
(8) Macaulay, N., U.S. Patent 3,016,308 (1962).
(9) Hall, H.S., and Hinkes, T.M., "Microencapsulation Processes and Applications", Vandegaer, J. E., editor, P. 145, Plenum Press, New York (1974).
(10) Vandegaer, J. E., U.S. Patent 3,577,515 (1971)
(11) Scher, H. B., Great Britain Patent 1,371,179 (1975).
(12) Brynko, C., U.S. Patent 2,969,330 (1961).
(13) Goodwin, J. T., and Somerville, G. R., "Microencapsulation Processes and Applications", Vandegaer, J. E., editor, P 155, Plenum Press, New York (1974).
(14) Berger, B. B., Miller, C. D., and Langer, G., U.S. Patent 3,208,951 (1965).
(15) Fanger, G. O., "Microencapsulation Processes and Applications", Vandegaer, J. E., editor, P 1, Plenum Press, New York (1974).
(16) Ivy, E. E., J. of Econ. Ent. (1972), 65, 473-474.
(17) Chem. and Eng. News, March 17, 1975, P 5.
(18) Plimmer, J. R., Bierl, B. A., DeVilbiss, E. D. and Smith, B. L., "Proceedings of the 1976 International Controlled Release Pesticide Symposium", Akron, Ohio.
(19) Markin, G. P., and Hill, S.O., J. of Econ. Ent. (1971), 64, 193-196.
(20) Rarn, E. S., and Jackson, R. D., J. of Econ. Ent. (1966), 59, 620-622.

13

Effects of Wall Parameters on the Release of Active Ingredients from Microencapsulated Insecticides

J. R. LOWELL, JR. and W. H. CULVER

Pennwalt Corp., 1630 E. Shaw Ave., Suite 179, Fresno, Calif. 93710

C. B. DeSAVIGNY

Pennwalt Corp., P. O. Box 3608, Bryan, Tex. 77801

Application of Pennwalt microencapsulation technology to methyl parathion has produced the first commercial microencapsulated pesticide, PENNCAP-M® Insecticide. In the course of our encapsulation development programs a substantial body of information has been collected regarding the effects of various wall parameters on release rates of microencapsulated formulations.

The polymer system used in preparation of PENNCAP-M is a crosslinked nylon-type polymer produced from sebacoyl chloride, ethylenediamine (EDA), diethylenetriamine (DETA), and polymethylenepolyphenylisocyanate (PAPI®). The active ingredient, diacid chloride and PAPI form a homogeneous mixture, which is dispersed in an aqueous medium. When brought into contact with an aqueous solution of the diamines, a shell of cross-linked nylon forms around each individual droplet. The product is typically formulated as an aqueous suspension, as with PENNCAP-M. While materials encapsulated may include liquids, solutions, suspensions, or solids, our efforts have been most successful with the two former categories. Encapsulation in similar polymers has produced effective insecticide formulations of Diazinon®, parathion, various pyrethroids, and malathion. In this paper some observations will be presented on the effects of capsule wall thickness, crosslinking, and acid chlorides on release rates of active ingredients.

Ivy[1] has previously reported on the reduction in mammalian toxicity and the extension of insecticidal activity resulting from encapsulation of methyl parathion. As presently marketed, PENNCAP-M is at least 6 times less toxic orally and 12 times less toxic dermally than emulsifiable concentrate formu-

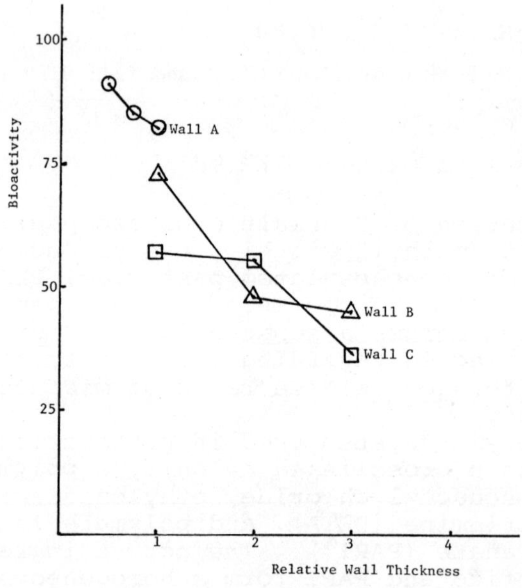

Figure 1. Effect of wall thickness on bioactivity of encapsulated parathion

lations of methyl parathion, on an active ingredient basis. Insecticidal activity is extended, up to 2½ times, depending on the crop and weather conditions.

DeSavigny and Ivy[2] have reported further on the Pennwalt microencapsulation process, revising the toxicology figures as production experience was obtained. Additional insect control reports confirmed the greater residual activity of PENNCAP-M as compared with EC formulations.

We have also reported on the use of PENNCAP-M for effective insect control on tobacco plants[3], and on the economics of microencapsulation as demonstrated by our experience with PENNCAP-M[4]. Koestler[5] has proposed a mechanism for the action of microencapsulated herbicides and insecticides, suggesting that the high number of particles, close particle spacing, and high local concentrations of toxicant are responsible for the effectiveness of the microencapsulated products.

During development of a new microencapsulated pesticides in our laboratories, candidate preparations are screened by means of a bioassay technique. The bioassay consists of spraying a suitable surface, usually bean foliage or cardboard, with a standard amount of the insecticide. The surface is then infested at suitable intervals with insects, generally crickets. Percent mortality is determined as a function of time after spraying. Corrected percent mortality figures for the duration of the test are averaged, giving a "Bioactivity" figure which approaches 100 for a material which is insecticidally active and persists for the duration of the test. Low bioactivity results most often indicate a rapid release and low persistence, but occasionally a formulation will produce a low percent mortality which persists for the duration of the test, indicating very slow release.

The thickness of the capsule wall can be estimated by simple geometry calculations to be directly proportional to the percentage of polymer-forming ingredients in the formulation. For any formulation, then, the "percent wall" can be represented as a relative wall thickness. In Figure 1, the bioactivity of parathion encapsulated in three different wall systems is depicted as a function of wall thickness. It is readily apparent that in each case the bioactivity dropped as the wall thickness increased. In the case of Wall A, in particular, the data showed that the percent mortality was increasing with time for all three wall thicknesses, indicating that the low bioactivity for this wall was due to very slow release.

In Figure 2, it can be seen that for Diazinon encapsulated in Wall D, bioactivity on foliage increased with increasing wall thickness until a plateau was reached. When tested in soil, however, the same formulation showed increases in bioactivity with increasing wall thickness until a peak was reached, after which the bioactivity decreased. Foliar bioactivity with malathion encapsulated in Wall D increased with increasing wall thickness. In Figure 3, results for encapsulated methyl parathion showed an insensitivity to wall thickness when encapsulated in Wall D. Another major factor influencing the release of active ingredient from capsules is crosslinking. In Figure 4, the data obtained showed a peak in bioactivity at 25% crosslinking for Wall E, using bollworms as the test insect. The increased bioactivity in this crosslinking study was associated with lower release rates.

DeGennaro et al.[6] have shown that the release of sodium pentobarbital increased with increasing crosslinking by increasing proportions of DETA. The increase was attributed to increasing porosity as the preparation became more highly crosslinked. It should be noted, however, that their studies utilized an ionic active ingredient, while our preparations have used relatively nonpolar organic materials. Crosslinking in their system was achieved with a polyfunctional amine, while in ours, a polyfunctional isocyanate is the principal source of crosslinking.

Effects of the identity of the acid chloride have not been extensively investigated in our laboratories. As shown in Figure 5, the bioactivity varied with the chain length of the dicarboxylic acid. In Wall F, as shown, the bioactivity was lowest with azelaoyl chloride, while adipoyl and sebacoyl chloride both gave significantly greater activity in this wall formulation.

In conclusion, the data presented here have shown that bioactivity varies in an irregular manner with increasing wall thickness and increasing crosslinking. The acid chloride chosen also affected activity, but testing has been insufficient to draw any conclusions. It must thus be concluded, then, that producing an optimum encapsulated pesticide formulation by the Pennwalt process still requires an empirical approach. For each product which has reached the field development stage, a painstaking laboratory investigation of each of these variables

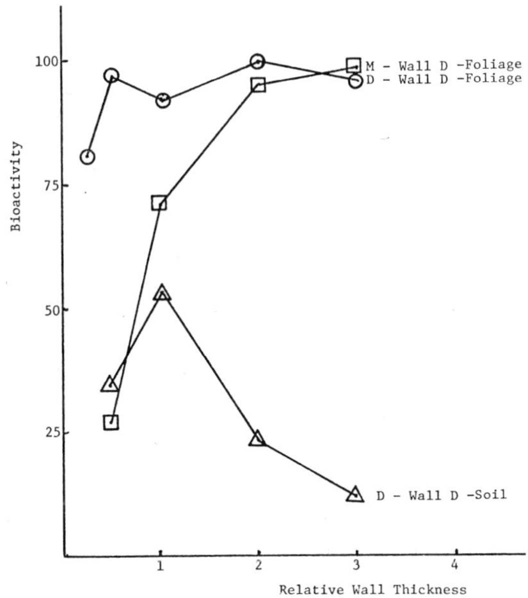

Figure 2. Effect of wall thickness on bioactivity of encapsulated Diazinon (D) and malathion (M)

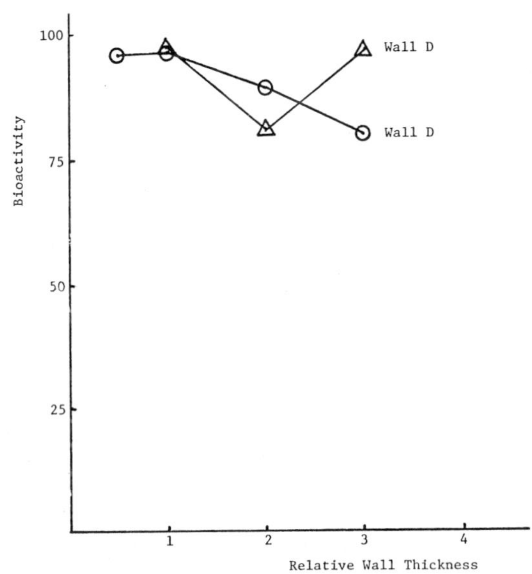

Figure 3. Effect of wall thickness on bioactivity of encapsulated methyl parathion

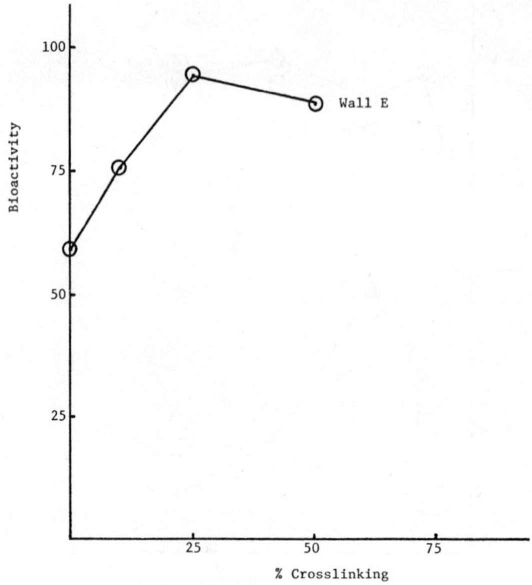

Figure 4. Effect of cross-linking on bioactivity of encapsulated methyl parathion

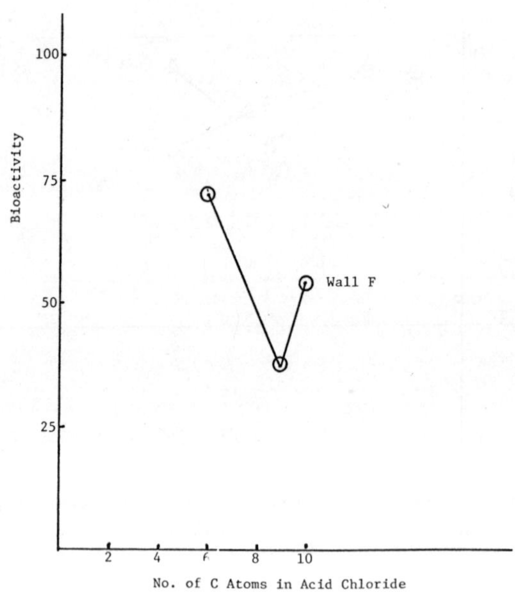

Figure 5. Effect of acid chloride chain length on bioactivity of encapsulated parathion

has been necessary.

One aspect of the effect of crosslinking is worth noting here. With regard to the suggestion of DeGennaro et al. that the effect of increasing crosslinking in their capsule formulations increased the release rate by increasing porosity, we generally have found the opposite effect with the relatively nonpolar pesticides which we have encapsulated, when crosslinking was effected by a polyfunctional isocyanate. It may be that the effects observed with increasing amounts of polyfunctional isocyanate relate to changes in the solvent properties of the capsule wall polymer, altering the solubility of the diffusing substance in the wall, and thus changing its diffusion characteristics. Unless affected by swelling or hydration effects, the effects of changes in microporosity should be similar in direction for ionic or nonionic materials. If the effect of the polymer composition is to alter the solubility of the encapsulated material in the polymer, then opposite effects for ionic and nonpolar species, as observed here, might be expected. We offer this as a working hypothesis deserving of further study.

PAPI is a trademark of Upjohn
Diazinon is a trademark of Ciba-Geigy

Literature Cited

1. E. E. Ivy, J. Econ. Entomol., 65(2), 473 (1972).
2. C. B. DeSavigny and E. E. Ivy, in J. E. Vandagaer, Editor, "Microencapsulation: Processes and Applications," Plenum Publishing Corp.
3. J. R. Lowell, Jr. and J. L. Frizzell, Reprints of Papers from the Symposium "Chemical Requirements of the Tobacco Industry," 169th Meeting of the American Chemical Society, Philadelphia, PA, April, 1975.
4. J. R. Lowell, Jr. and J. J. Murnighan, Reprints of Papers from the Symposium "Economics and Market Opportunities for Controlled Release Products," 172nd Meeting of the American Chemical Society, San Francisco, CA, August, 1976.
5. R. C. Koestler, in N. F. Cardarelli, Editor, "Proceedings 1976 Controlled Release Pesticide Symposium," Akron, OH, September, 1976.
6. M. DeGennaro, et al., in D. R. Paul and F. W. Harris, Ed., "Controlled Release Polymeric Formulations," ACS Symposium Series, American Chemical Society, Washington, D.C., 1976, pp. 195-207.

14

The Effect of Some Variables on the Controlled Release of Chemicals from Polymeric Membranes

AGIS F. KYDONIEUS

Hercon Products Group, Herculite Protective Fabrics Corp.,
1107 Broadway, New York, N.Y. 10010

Controlled release technology is the adaptation of permeation processes to the dispensing of toxic, volatile, unstable and other chemicals. Nature, Naivete and ingenuity have provided a number of well known examples of permeation controlled processes.

Some well known processes which depend on permeation are: respiration, osmosis, and the "bloom" or "patina" on grapes and other fruit. Inspection of these examples reveal that gases, liquids, and solids may be observed to pass through various membrane materials.

The manner in which permeation takes place through the HERCON® laminated polymeric membrane system and the factors affecting such permeation will be discussed.

1. The HERCON Dispensing System

A schematic cross-section of a typical HERCON laminated membrane structure is shown in Figure 1. The specially formulated inner layer, which behaves as the reservoir, contains dissolved insecticide or other active agent which then migrates continually, due to imbalance of chemical potential, through one or more initially inert outer layers to the surface, rendering it biologically or physico-chemically active. At the surface, the insecticide is removed by volatilization, thermal or ultraviolet degradation, alkaline or acid hydrolysis, or mechanically by humans, insects, rainfall, wind or other agents.

The construction and composition of the laminated insecticidal membranes vary , of course, with the active agent used, release rate and effective life span desired. However, materials containing from 0.5 to 40%, by weight, active agent have been successfully prepared and have been shown by laboratory and field tests to be efficacious in a number of applications (1, 2).

2. The Mathematics of Transport

The class of membranes used with the HERCON technology is the nonporous, homogeneous polymeric films. These membranes are usually referred to as solution-diffusion membranes. Silicone rubber, polyethylene, polyvinylchloride and nylon films are typical examples.

The penetrant is able to pass through the membrane material in the absence of pores or holes by a process of absorption, solution, diffusion down a gradient of thermo-dynamic activity and desorption. The process of permeation thus is divisible into a number of independent processes governed primarily by Henry's law and Fick's law (3, 4).

Transport of active chemical from the reservoir through the barrier membrane is governed by Fick's first law:

$$J = -D \frac{dC_m}{dx} \qquad [1]$$

where J is the flux in g/cm^2-sec, C_m is the concentration of permeant in the membrane in g/cm^3, dC_m/dx is the gradient in concentration, and D is the diffusion coefficient of the permeant in the membrane in cm^2/sec.

(a) The Steady State. As shown in Figure 2, the concentration just inside the membrane surface can be related to the concentration in the reservoir C by the expressions:

$$C_m(0) = KC_{(0)} \text{ at the upstream surface } (x = 0)$$
$$C_m(1) = KC_{(1)} \text{ at the downstream surface } (x = 1) \qquad [2]$$

here, K is a distribution coefficient and is analogous to the familiar liquid-liquid partition coefficient. In Figure 2, for purposes of illustration, it has been assumed that the distribution is less than unity for barrier membrane I, and more than unity for membrane II. Throughout the following, we will assume diffusion coefficients and distribution coefficients to be constant. This is a safe assumption for most polymer-permeant systems. Thus, in the steady state, Equation [1] can be integrated to give:

$$J = D \frac{C_m(0) - C_m(1)}{1} = D \frac{\Delta C_m}{1} \qquad [3]$$

where 1 is the thickness of the membrane. Since the concentration within the membrane is usually not known, Equation [3] is frequently

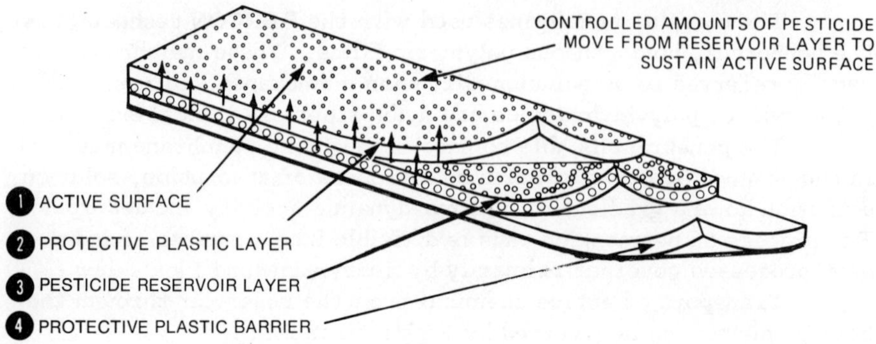

Figure 1. Schematic of Hercon laminated controlled release structure

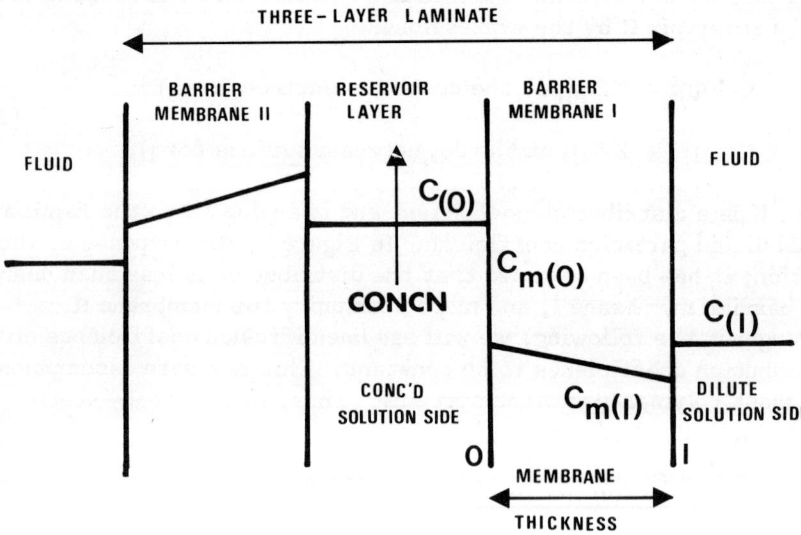

Figure 2. Schematic of the concentration gradient across a three-layer laminate

written:

$$J = \frac{dM_t}{dt} = \frac{DK\Delta C}{1} \qquad [4]$$

where M_t is the mass of agent released, $\frac{dM_t}{dt}$ is the steady state release rate at time t and ΔC is the difference in concentration $(C_{(0)} - C_{(1)})$ between the reservoir concentration and the fluid concentration adjacent to the barrier membrane.

It is significant to note that the rate of release is proportional to diffusivity (a kinetic constant) and to distribution coefficient (a thermodynamic constant). Equation [4] can be integrated between the limits:

$$\begin{aligned} M_t &= 0 \quad t = 0 \\ M_t &= M_t \quad t = t \end{aligned} \qquad [5]$$

to give: $$M_t = \frac{ADK\Delta C_t}{1}$$

When the distribution coefficient between the reservoir layer and the barrier membrane is much smaller than unity, as is the case of membrane I in Figure 2, the system has excellent release kinetics and the release rate can be maintained constant for extended periods of time (pseudo-zero order delivery). Equation [5] is then governing the process and a straight line is obtained when the mass of agent released (M_t) is plotted against time (t). This is shown in Figure 3, with a polyvinyl chloride-polyester system.

(b) <u>The Unsteady State</u>. When the distribution coefficient between the reservoir layer and the barrier membrane is approximately unity, or larger than unity, as is the case with membrane II of Figure 2, the HERCON system will approximate the "dissolved system", i.e., the reservoir - barrier membrane system forms a single homogeneous polymeric film. The concentration in the reservoir will not remain constant but will fall continuously with time. The system remains continuously under unsteady state conditions and the mass of agent released varies as a function of time (first order delivery). The transport equations have been described by several investigators (5, 6, 7).

The two useful equations are the early time approximation, which holds over the initial portion of the curve:

$$\frac{M_t}{M_\infty} = 4\left(\frac{Dt}{\pi 1^2}\right)^{1/2} \quad 0 \leqslant \frac{M_t}{M} \leqslant 0.6 \qquad [6]$$

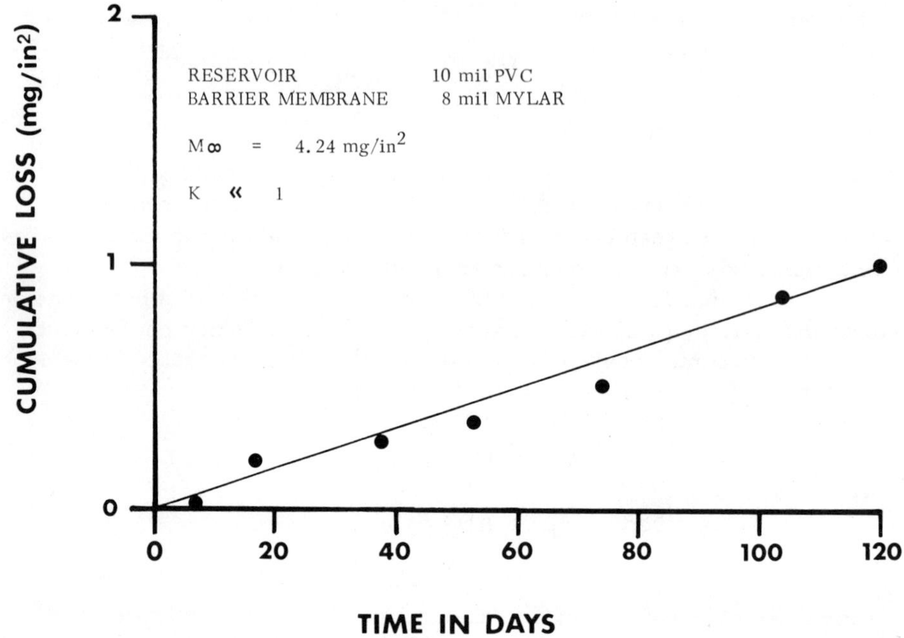

Figure 3. Release of fly repellent MGK R-874—reservoir-type system

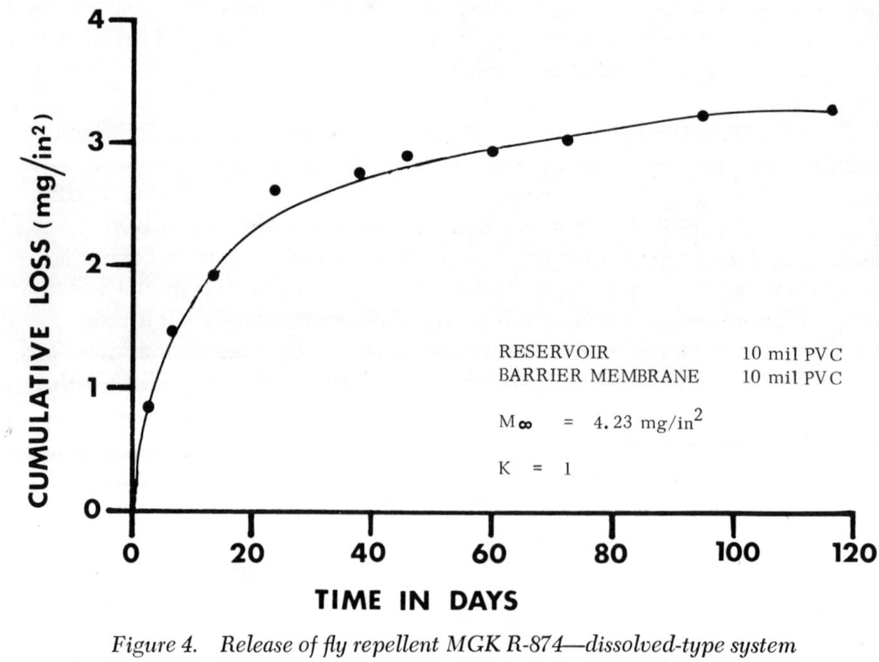

Figure 4. Release of fly repellent MGK R-874—dissolved-type system

and the late time approximation, which holds over the final portion of the release curve,

$$\frac{M_t}{M_\infty} = 1 - \frac{8}{\pi^2} \exp \frac{(-\pi^2 Dt)}{l^2} \quad 0.4 \leq \frac{M_t}{M} \leq 1.0 \qquad [7]$$

As it can be seen from equation [6], a plot of mass of agent released versus time will give a parabolic curve. This is the case for the PVC-PVC system shown in Figure 4. When the same data are plotted versus $(\text{time})^{1/2}$, a linear curve is obtained, (Figure 5), in accordance with Equation [6].

3. Factors Affecting the Release

Looking at equations [5], [6], and [7], it becomes apparent that the release of active ingredients from HERCON laminated membrane structures is controlled by molecular and structural factors. For a given combination of polymer structure and active agent where energy to free rotations, free volume, and intermolecular attractions are constant, at least two parameters are available to regulate the rate of transfer: reservoir concentration and membrane thickness.

Diffusivity D and reservoir/membrane distribution coefficient K are also directly proportional to the permeation rate. In polymers, diffusivity is strongly sensitive to the molecular weight of the diffusant and to the stiffness of the backbone of the polymeric membrane. Simply speaking, the diffusant molecule will have to reorient several segments of polymer chain to allow its passage from site to site. The higher the molecular weight, the more the segments that need to be reoriented for passage to be possible; and the stiffer the polymer (glassy and high crystallinity), the more difficult for its segments to undergo large reorientations. Therefore, variables that could affect the stiffness of polymer membranes such as co-diffusants that would soften, plasticize or partially dissolve the membrane would have an effect on diffusivity and permeation rate.

The reservoir/membrane distribution coefficient K can be estimated from the solubility parameter of the diffusant. Solubility parameters can be calculated using Hilderbrand's solubility theory. When the solubility parameter for the diffusant and polymer membrane is the same, the polymer will be soluble in the diffusant. The solubility parameters and dissolution are strongly affected by molecular weight and the chemical functionality of the molecule, i.e., hydrogen bonding and polarity. Like dissolves like is still a good rule of thumb.

I would like to take a few minutes now to discuss the effect

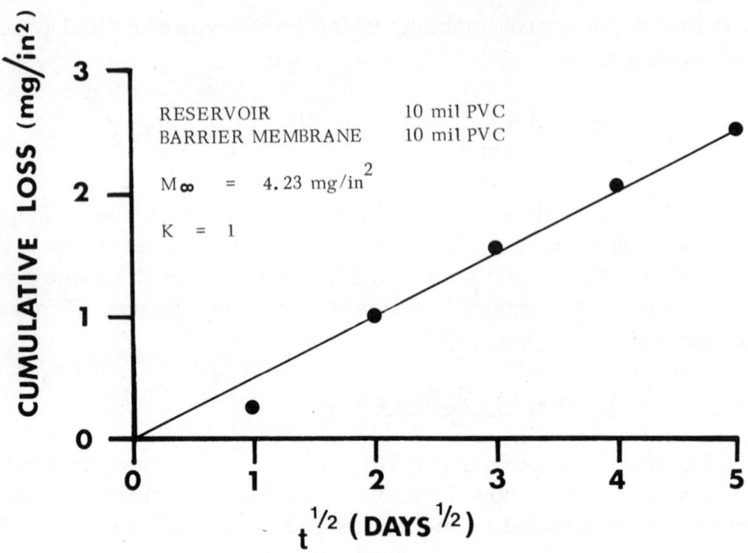

Figure 5. Release of fly repellent MGK R-874—dissolved-type system

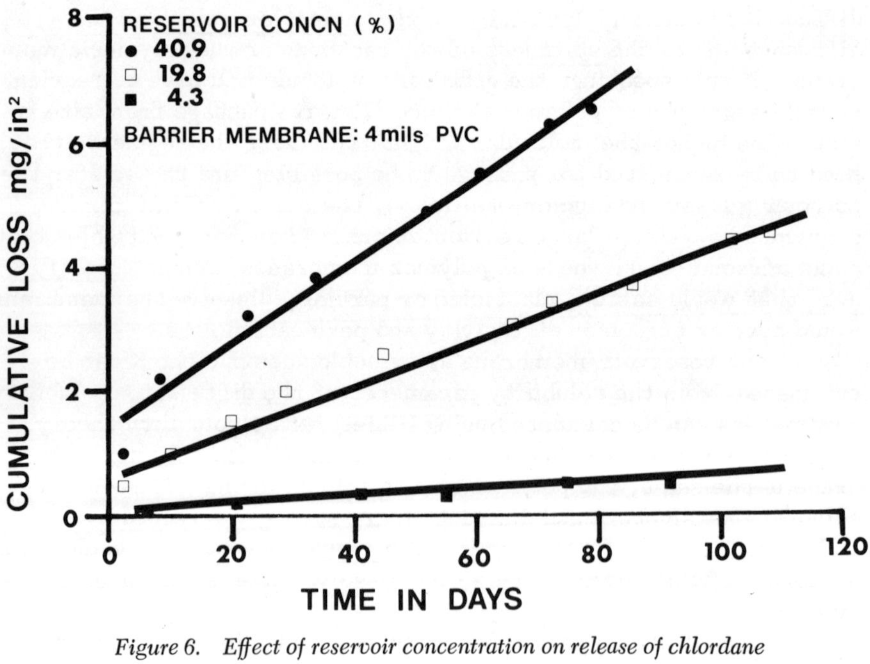

Figure 6. Effect of reservoir concentration on release of chlordane

of: 1) reservoir concentration, 2) membrane thickness, 3) polymer stiffness, 4) co-diffusants, 5) molecular weight of diffusant and 6) chemical functionality on the transport of active ingredients through HERCON laminated membranes. For purposes of illustration and simplicity in all examples that follow, the reservoir is made of flexible polyvinylchloride.

Reservoir Concentration. In Figures 6 and 7, the release of the pesticide chlordane and the insect repellent DEET are illustrated. In both cases, zero order release rates were obtained. A closer look indicates that doubling the concentration in the reservoir does not double the mass of agent released. This deviation is more pronounced at higher concentrations, presumably because the inter-molecular attraction of the diffusant molecules increase exponentially with concentration.

With the exception of these minor differences, the data in general terms follow equations [5] and [6].

Membrane Thickness. Both equations [5] and [6] indicate that the mass of agent released should be inversely proportional to the thickness of the membrane. This is shown to be the case with the repellent DEET and the pheromones dodecenyl acetate and Hexadecyl Acetate (Figures 8 and 9).

Polymer Stiffness. The distribution coefficient K for several polymer membranes of different backbone stiffness and PVC was studied, by adhering large reservoir layers of PVC to said membranes. The transport of active agent from the reservoir to the membrane was studied by separating the layers and determining the amount of active agent by chemical analysis. This is shown in Table A for the active agents: Captan-an antibacterial agent, Malathion-an insecticide, and Zineb-an agricultural fungicide. For all three agents, the amount transported into the membranes becomes progressively smaller, going from PVC to rigid vinyl, polypropylene, nylon and mylar, which also corresponds to increase in backbone stiffness.

Distribution coefficients were not calculated because 20 weeks after the experiments were initiated, it was not certain that equilibrium had been reached in most cases. The amount of active chemical transported with time for a few cases is shown in Table B.

In a second experiment, the diffusion into films of different backbone stiffness was monitored by the properties imparted to said films. The antibacterial agent, Captan, the germicide, vinazene, and the antistatic agent, Ethoquad, were used. The results, shown in Table C, indicate that the effectiveness of the films was, in general,

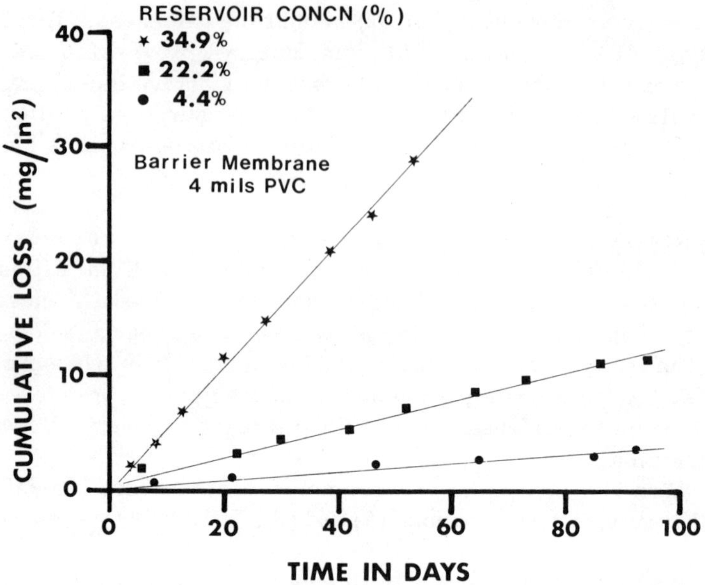

Figure 7. Effect of reservoir concentration on release of DEET

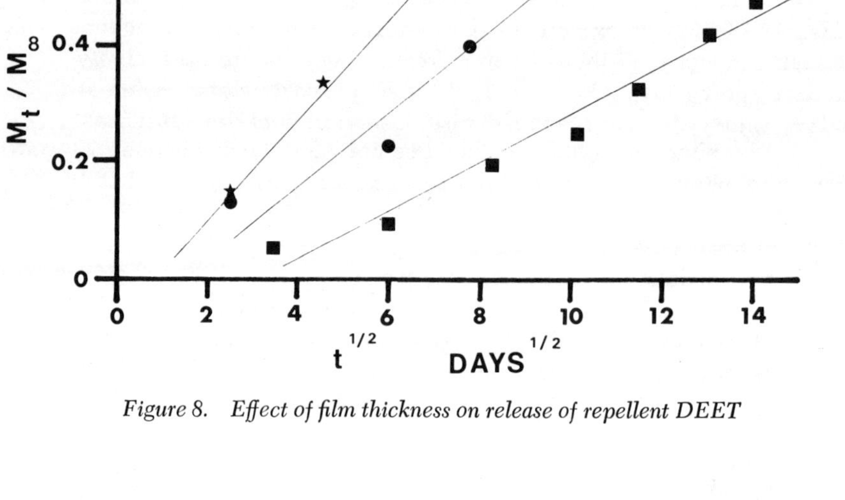

Figure 8. Effect of film thickness on release of repellent DEET

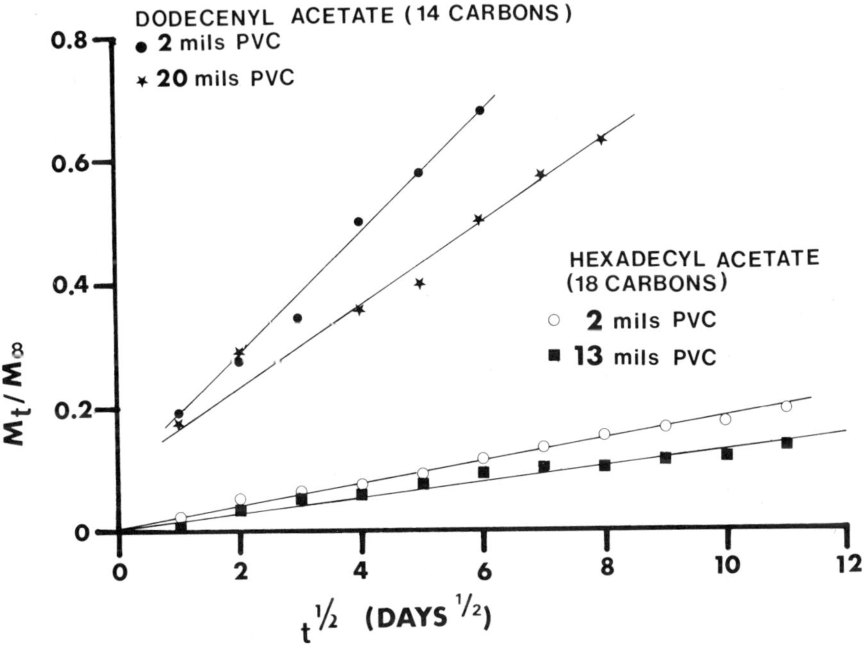

Figure 9. Effect of film thickness on mass of agent released

best for flexible PVC, followed by rigid PVC, acrylic, polyproplene, nylon and polyester. This order is the same as that of the dats shown in Table A, with effectiveness reduced as the backbone stiffness was increased.

Table A

Distribution of Active Agents between Flexible PVC and Polymer Increasing Backbone Stiffness

	ACTIVE AGENT TRANSPORTED (ppm)				
	Flex PVC[1]	Rigid PVC	Polyprop	Nylon	Polyester
Captan	250	109	36	3	0
Malathion	12000	9700	498	23	8
Zineb	1600	568	62	63	9

1 All Polymer films were 5 mils thick. The total amount of Captan, Malathion and Zineb in the system were 500, 24000 and 4000 ppm, respectively. Readings were taken 20 weeks after the initiation of Experiment.

Table B

Active Agent transported as a Function of Time (ppm)

	2 weeks	7 weeks	20 weeks
Malathion			
Rigid PVC	6300	9000	9700
Nylon	6	12	23
Polyprop	387	334	498
Captan			
Rigid PVC	29	55	109
Polyprop	1	26	36
Zineb			
Rigid PVC	303	619	568
Nylon	67	60	62

Co-diffusants. Chemical agents that are capable in altering the structure (e.g., stiffness) of a polymer would have a pronounced effect on the diffusion of active chemicals that are allowed to co-diffuse. These "carrier" materials must have the ability to swell, soften and/or dissolve the polymer matrix. A good example is the impartment of antistatic properties to nylon and polyester carpets by using the co-diffusants phenol and ethylene glycol phenyl ether, respectively (8). Table D shows that 3 fold and 100 fold improvements in antistatic resistivity can be obtained for nylon and polyester respectively by using the co-diffusants mentioned above.

Table C.

Property Improvement by Diffusion of Active Chemicals

	Flex PVC	Rigid PVC	Acrylic	Polyprop	Nylon	Polyester
Vinazene [germicide]	7.0[1]	12	-	15	0	0
Captan [antibacterial]	99.9+[2]	99.9+	88.2	97.8	42.3	48.2
Ethoquad [antistatic]	10000[3]	4200	2100	1100	420	73

[1] Zone of Inhibition in mm

[2] Reduction of bacteria over untreated control (NYS-63)

[3] Reduction in Surface Resistivity ($\frac{\text{Ohms}}{\text{sq}}$) over untreated control

Molecular Weight. The molecular weight of the diffusant is very important because it is directly related to the diffusivity. To investigate the effect of molecular weight on the transport through polymer membranes, five (5) insect pheromones were chosen. Although not exactly of the same homologous series, they were all acetates ranging from 12 carbon atoms to 20 carbon atoms. The release through a 2 mil flexible polyvinylchloride membrane is shown in Figure 10. The strong influence of molecular weight is apparent from this graph, with sharp decreases in release rate as the molecular weight increased from 198 to 310 in steps of 28 units.

Chemical Functionality. Like dissolves like is equally applicable in the polymer area. Dissolution of the polymer matrix by the diffusing molecules is important in the transport process because it increases the value of the distribution coefficient. To study this variable, two sets of pheromones with 16 and 20 carbon atoms, respectively, were investigated. The results are depicted in Figures 11 and 12 and show that functionality has a substantial effect on the

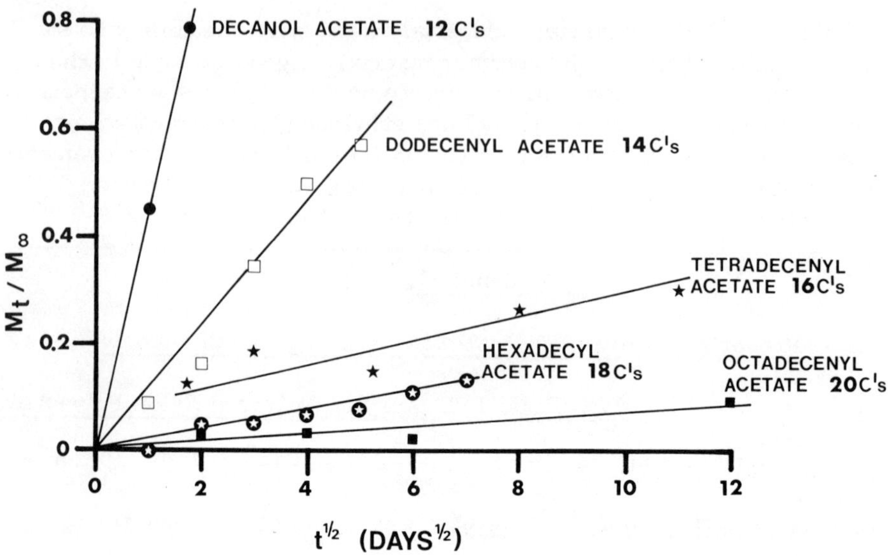

Figure 10. Effect of molecular weight on mass of agent released

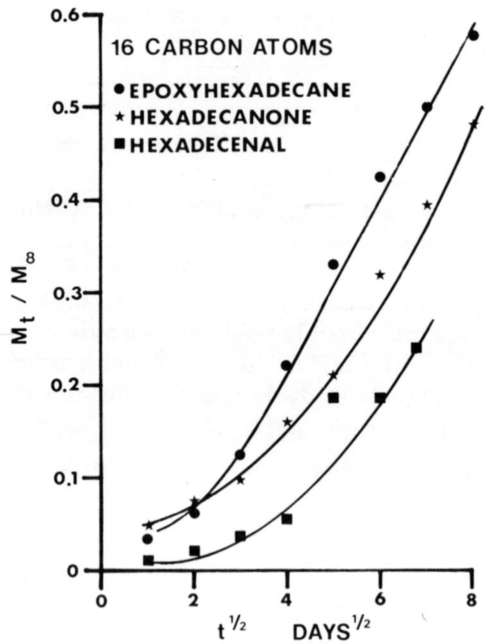

Figure 11. Effect of functionality on release rate

Table D.

The Effect of Co-Diffusants on the Antistatic Properties of Carpets

CARPET FIBER	Antistatic Agent	Co-Diffusant	Active Agent Concentration	Volume Resistivity (ohms)
NYLON (Bigelow)	Advastat 50	Phenol	14.7	7.0×10^8
	Advastat 50	None	14.8	2.2×10^9
	None	None	None	1.1×10^{11}
POLYESTER (DuPont)	Advastat 50	Dowanol EPh	17.6	7.0×10^8
	Advastat 50	None	16.9	8.0×10^{10}
	None	None	None	1.1×10^{11}

Reservoir Polymer Matrix: VULCANOL 5023

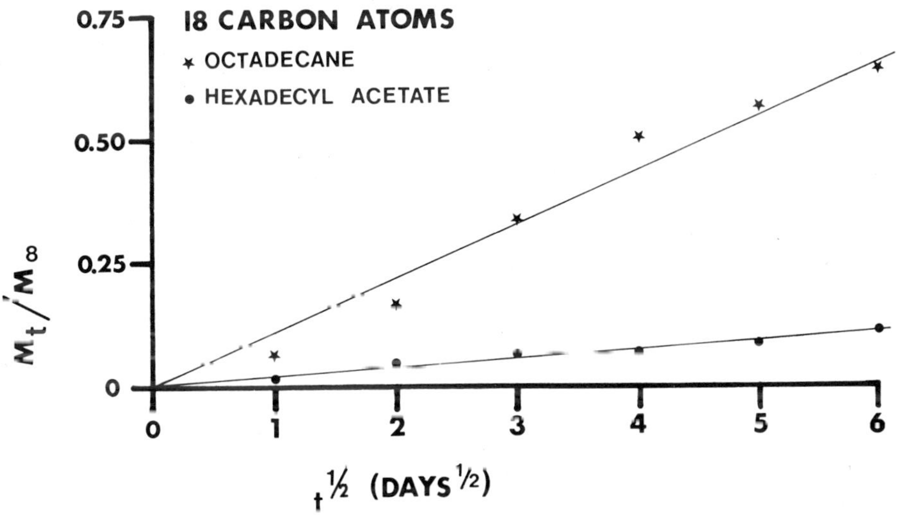

Figure 12. Effect of functionality on release rate

Table E

Some Commercial Products Using the HERCON technology

Product	Membrane I	Membrane II	Function
STAPH-CHEK®	4 mil PVC	4 mil PVC	Antibacterial hospital fabric
INSECTAPE®	2 mil mylar	5 mil PVC	Roach control
LURE-N-KILL™ FLYTAPE			House fly control
Attractant	2 mil mylar	8 mil PVC	
Pesticide	2 mil PVC	2 mil PVC	
SCENTSTRIP™ I	2 mil mylar	5 mil PVC	Air freshener
SCENTSTRIP™ II	cloth	cloth	(consumer)
SCENTCOIL™	vinyl	vinyl	Air freshener (industrial)
LURETAPE™			
Disparlure	2 mil vinyl	2 mil vinyl	monitoring gypsy moth
Gossyplure	5 mil vinyl	5 mil vinyl	monitoring pink bollworm
Orfralure	6 mil acrylic	6 mil acrylic	Control of oriental fruit moth
Multilure	mylar	mylar	Control of elm bark beetle
Grandlure	16 mil rigid PVC	16 mil rigid PVC	Monitoring of boll weevil

release rate. As a matter of fact, octadecane had a much faster release rate than hexadecyl acetate as well as all of the 16 carbon atom pheromones shown in Figure 11.

4. Flexibility of the HERCON Process.

It has been shown that a large variety of factors affect the release through polymer films. The HERCON process with its flexibility in controlling release by varying membrane polymer thickness, membrane polymer matrix, reservoir polymer matrix and diffusant concentration as well as co-diffusants is capable in controlling the release of chemical agents to produce consumer and industrial products with improved properties, inexpensively.

Table E describes some of the commercial products that use the HERCON technology. Thickness and type of films are given for each product. The reservoir layer which is perhaps the most important aspect of the technology varies from product to product and it is of proprietary nature.

Our company is looking forward to the continuous expansion of the market for controlled release products and we are aggressively exploring new product applications using the technology mentioned herein.

LITERATURE CITED

(1) Kydonieus et al., "Marketing and Economic Considerations for HERCON Consumer and Industrial Controlled Release Products", ACS Proceedings-Chemical Marketing and Economics Division-1976, pp. 140-165.
(2) Kydonieus et al., "Controlled Release of Pheromones through Multi-layered Polymeric Dispensers", ACS Symposium Series 33, pps. 283-294, 1976.
(3) Crank, J. and G.S. Park, ed. "Diffusion in Polymers" Academic Press, N.Y.
(4) Richards, R.W., "The Permeability of Polymers to Gases, Vapours and Liquids; ERDE (Ministry of Defense) Tech. Report No. 135, March 1973, NTIS AD-767 627.
(5) Baker, R.W. and H.K. Lonsdale, "Controlled Release of Biologically Active Agents, A.C. Tanquary and R.E. Lacey (Eds.), Plenum Press, N.Y., 1974.
(6) Crank, J., "The Mathematics of Diffusion", Oxford University Press, London, 1956.
(7) Barrer, R.M., Diffusion in Polymers", Academic Press, London, 1968.
(8) Kydonieus, et.al., U.S. Patent 3,961,117 (1976).

15

Controlled Release of Pheromone in the Gypsy Moth Program

J. R. PLIMMER, B. A. BIERL, and R. E. WEBB

Beltsville Agricultural Research Center, U.S. Department of Agriculture, Beltsville, Md. 20705

C. P. SCHWALBE

Animal and Plant Health Inspection Service, U.S. Department of Agriculture, Otis Air Force Base, Mass. 02542

Progress in development and practical application of behavior-modifying chemicals has continued since research on the control of the gypsy moth, Lymantria Dispar (L.) and other insects with behavior-modifying chemicals was summarized in 1975 (1), and there has been considerable effort towards obtaining a greater understanding of the relationship between pheromone composition and the behavior associated with chemical stimuli (2). This is particularly true of the application of behavior-modifying chemicals in attempts to disrupt insect mating and thus to control pest populations. This appealing concept has many potential advantages. It is quite specific, and the quantity of material used (a few grams per hectare) is so small that its impact on the environment and on non-target species should be minimal. Pheromones generally show very low toxicity towards living organisms (3). Most insect pheromones contain only carbon, hydrogen and oxygen, and they would not be expected to pollute the environment because they are readily biodegradable. Their value for detection and survey of insect pest infestations has already been demonstrated. If pheromones can be applied effectively they should play an important role in the management of economic species, and there are many situations in which pheromones might be used with advantage to supplement conventional insecticides.

Sex pheromones are not expected to be effective in reducing insect populations in heavily infested areas (4); it is therefore important to define by experiment the population level at which mating can be prevented.

It must also be possible to monitor the progress of attempts to disrupt mating throughout the period of mating activity. When dealing with agricultural crops, economic benefit may be measured by reduction of crop damage in a treated plot compared with that observed in a control. However, it is often very difficult to define economic benefit that results from application to forest insects unless valuable timber resources are suffering attack.

In addition to establishing methods of defining effectiveness of pheromone treatments in terms of population reduction, we must also determine when and how pheromones should be used. These questions must be answered by considering the behavior of the insect and by investigating the physico-chemical characteristics of potential methods of delivering the pheromone.

The Gypsy Moth [Lymantria dispar (L.)]: Role of the Sex Pheromone

Since the insect was introduced into the U.S. in 1868 or 1869, gypsy moth infestations have spread over the greater portion of the northeastern United States where they have defoliated large areas of forest and shade trees (5). The gypsy moth is also found in temperate areas throughout the world from North Africa to Japan. In the late summer, the adult female deposits an egg mass that may contain 300 to 800 eggs. Larvae emerging from these egg masses early the following May consume large quantities of foliar material. (In Japan, male larvae consume 700 to 1100 cm^2 and females 110 to 1800 cm^2 of leaves) (6). The fully developed larvae pupate and emerge as adult moths from late June to August, depending on local climate. Mating activity extends over a period of 6 to 8 weeks.

The female does not normally fly and attracts the male for mating purposes by emitting a pheromone. Although other stimuli, such as visual cues, are important in mating, the sex pheromone of the moth (disparlure, cis-7,8-epoxy-2-methyloctadecane) acts as a powerful attractant. Pheromone emission follows a diel periodicity (7). The females become attractive after 0900 hours and remain attractive until about 2000 hours. Male response closely follows this periodicity: peak response occurs between 0900 and 1500 hours.

In our efforts to disrupt mating, synthetic racemic disparlure was used because it could be manufactured for a reasonable cost and has proved to be a good attractant. However, in 1974 Japanese workers synthesized the two optically active enantiomers of disparlure and found that the (+) enantiomer (7R,8S-epoxy-2-methyloctadecane) was much more effective as a trapping agent than the opposite enantiomer (8). Other experiments have confirmed its attractiveness (9,10,11). Therefore, it seems likely that the (+) enantiomer is identical to the naturally occurring pheromone. However, the enantiomers have so far been available only in milligram quantities (8,12), and their future impact on mating disruption experiments cannot be assessed until the possibilities of an economical synthesis have been explored.

Mating Disruption: Use of Pheromone Formulations

The suggestion was made in 1960 (13) that the artificial release of insect sex pheromones into the atmosphere would interfere with the process of mate-finding and thus with the mating process. The antennal sensillae of the male function as very specific receptors for the pheromone emitted by the female. The receptor sites are activated by specific chemicals or blends of chemicals, thus ensuring that communication is limited to members of the same species. However, the study of chemical stimuli alone is inadequate for understanding the complex phenomena associated with mating. Superimposed on the chemical communication system of individual insect species is a variety of behavioral and physiological characteristics. Techniques for disruption of mating must be based not only on the use of chemical formulations but also on knowledge of the behavior and biology of the target insect.

The design of chemical formulations demands that consideration be given to the interplay of many complex variables. Most attractant pheromones are relatively expensive chemicals, many of which readily decompose on exposure to light or air. Treatment of areas infested by the gypsy moth should be limited to one or two applications if pheromone use is to be economical. Fortunately, pheromones possess extremely high biological activity and, if they can be used to maximum effect, applications of only a few grams per acre should be adequate to achieve mating disruption (14).

The requirements for a formulation that will release sufficient pheromone to permeate the air and achieve disruption of mating over a prolonged period are quite exacting. For example, a constant release rate over a long period seems desirable. Some formulations show apparent zero order rate of emission (i.e., constant release rate independent of pheromone loading) if the reservoir of pheromone is so large that only a small fraction only is emitted over a long period (15). However, to reduce the amount of expensive ingredient used, we designed types of formulation that were intended to release the major portion of their loading of pheromone over the flight season of the male gypsy moth (6-8 weeks).

Formulation performance is affected by environmental factors such as temperature. Pheromone release rate from the formulation should be characterized by a positive temperature coefficient, because the mating activity of the gypsy moth is at its most intense at mid-day and during the afternoon. Diurnal temperature variations will favor the desired performance. Pheromone emission will increase as the temperature increases during the day, whereas very little of the pheromone will be released during the cooler period throughout the night. However a formulation possessing these characteristics would probably be less effective against insects that showed maximum mating activity in the dark.

Controlled release formulations

Controlled release formulations have proved their worth as a source of pheromone for use in traps. The USDA detection and survey trap (delta trap) (Figure 1) consists of an open-ended cardboard tube of triangular cross section (16). The interior is coated with a sticky material and contains a dispenser that slowly releases disparlure, thus providing a bait. The dispenser currently in use (the Hercon ® dispenser, manufactured by the Health Chem. Corp., New York, N.Y. 10010 [1/]) is a three-layer plastic laminate (17). The two outer plastic layers cover an inner layer impregnated with disparlure. We have determined the effects of loading, wall thickness, and temperature on the rate of emission of disparlure from this dispenser (18). A dispenser of 6 mils thickness containing 6 mg of disparlure emitted 0.24 μg of pheromone/hr at 80°F in a constant flow of air of 100 ml/min. An increase of 10°F almost doubled the rate of emission. Although the rate of emission should be dependent on the weight of lure present, in 20 days only 115 μg was lost at 80°F. Since this is a very small fraction of the total lure content, we may regard the emission rate as constant during the period of male flight.

By contrast, if we wish to use a broadcast formulation to disrupt mating, more efficient use of the expensive pheromone is preferable. In addition, unnecessary increases in the environmental burden of synthetic biologically active compounds are undesirable. It must be borne in mind that the amount of active ingredient applied per hectare is irrelevant in terms of our objective when we use pheromones to permeate the air; the amount of material released by the formulation during the period of mating is more significant, and this quantity is dependent on the type of the formulation. However, for comparison during field trials we maintained the rate of application constant at 20 grams of disparlure per hectare (8 g/acre).

Several formulation types were selected for laboratory evaluation. Within each formulation type, possible modifications can increase factorially the number of candidates for testing.

In 1975, large scale field tests were restricted to microencapsulated formulations. In 1976, on the basis of laboratory results several other formulations were included in the field program (Table I).

1/ Mention of a manufacturer or a proprietary product does not imply endorsement by the USDA.

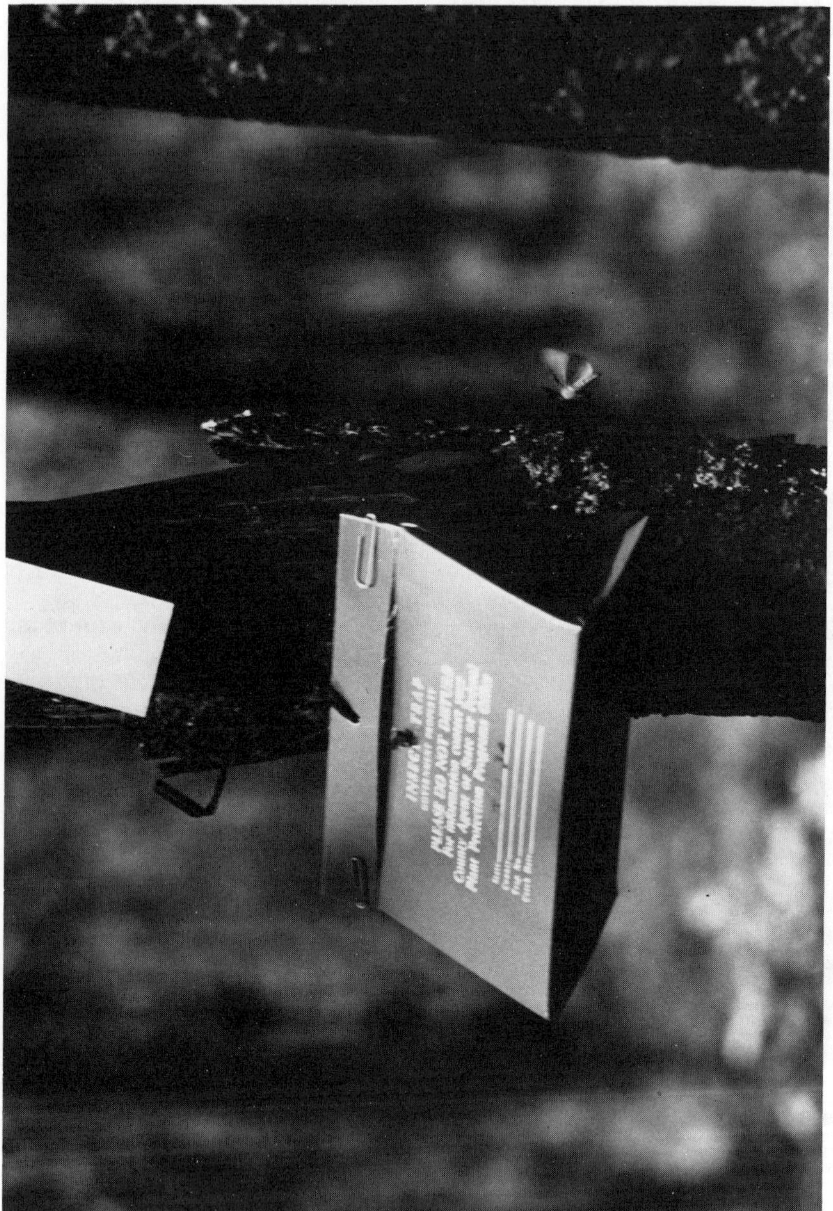

Figure 1. A USDA *detection and survey trap (delta trap)*

TABLE I

Formulations Used in Field Testing

Formulation designation	Manufacturer	% Lure in Particles	Particle size (μ)
1976-NCR-2	National Cash Register	2	50-250
1976-NCR-4	National Cash Register	3/4 : 2 1/4 : 10	50-250
1976-NCR-10	National Cash Register	10	50-250
1975-NCR-2	National Cash Register	2	50-400
Stauffer	Stauffer Chemical Co.	3/4 : 2 1/4 : 10	10-40
MGK	McLaughlin Gormley King Co.	2	100-200
Conrel	Albany International Co.	30	Fibers

Microencapsulated formulations based on gelatin-walled capsules (National Cash Register Corp., Dayton, Ohio), and on polyurea-walled capsules (Stauffer Chemical Co., Richmond, Calif.) were examined. Also tested were a "matrix" formulation (McLaughlin, Gormley, King and Co., Minneapolis, Minn.) and hollow fibers containing disparlure (Conrel, Albany International Co., Norwood, Mass.). All the formulations with the exception of the Conrel hollow fiber type, for which special equipment was necessary, were suitable for conventional spray application from aircraft. They were applied from Spraying System No. 8010 tips on spray boom nozzles.

Formulations for Broadcast Application

Previous experience (19) gave a good indication of the types of formulation that might be expected to perform well in the field. Among the candidates selected for testing were various types of microcapsules. Although the behavior of encapsulated pheromones would appear to be predictable *a priori*, we learned by experiment that their longevity in the field was greatly affected by environmental factors.

The rate at which the pheromone is released was affected not only by the pheromone loading and the chemical composition of the capsule wall and the other components of the formulation, but also by humidity, temperature and sunlight. Microcapsules of different wall permeability or size can be made by changing the manufacturing process. Because changes in disparlure content can affect release rate, disparlure was encapsulated at two different concentrations (2% and 10%) in solution. The designation 2% and 10% refer to the concentration of disparlure in the solvent; the Stauffer and 4% NCR formulations comprised a 75:25 mixture of the

2% and 10% materials.

The release rate of disparlure from a microcapsule should undergo approximately exponential decay as its concentration decreases. In practice, spray application of microcapsules is sometimes followed by a 'burst' of pheromone, which may possibly be ascribed to loss from a capsular membrane initially saturated with disparlure. After the initial burst, the slope of the plot of release rate versus time decreases. Some microcapsules, observed under a microscope, appeared to lose their contents rapidly and become distorted. This collapse appeared to be related to high relative humidity.

In consequence, we examined the effect of some of these variables in a series of laboratory tests before field evaluation. These tests were carried out as follows:

1) Preliminary Screening: Samples of the candidate formulations were applied to microscope slides and aged outdoors in slide boxes hung under a canopy to protect them from rain but not from wind and temperature changes. Other samples were aged indoors. The rate of emission of pheromone was measured periodically at constant temperature in the apparatus previously described (20). The amount of pheromone remaining in the formulation was also determined as a function of exposure time. These two measurements did not always give the same evaluation. The emission rate provided a better guide to performance than measurement of residual pheromone, since we found that some microencapsulated formulations ceased emitting disparlure even though a substantial amount of the pheromone was still present in the capsules.

2) Evaluation of Sticker: Microencapsulated formulations contain capsules suspended in water with a surfactant and a thickening agent (usually hydroxyethylcellulose) to stabilize the suspension. Microcapsules deposited onto foliage are rapidly washed off by rain or dislodged by the effect of wind; therefore stickers are added to the formulations to ensure that the capsules adhere tightly to the foliage. Larger capsules seem to be dislodged more readily than the smaller ones, and the choice of capsule size was influenced by this knowledge. Stickers were tested in the laboratory by applying the formulation, including the sticker, to foliage and allowing it to dry for 1 to 2 hours. A spray of water was applied to determine whether the formulation was readily washed off.

Because stickers can form adhesive films, they reduce the rate of emission of pheromone from the microcapsules and, in effect, prolong the effectiveness of the formulation. As further evaluation, the emission rates of the formulations were measured with and without addition of sticker.

3) Effect of Environmental Conditions: In the field, formulations are usually exposed to severe weathering. Wind, sun, and rain will have considerable influence in decreasing the lifetime of a microencapsulated pheromone formulation. Therefore, we measured the lifetime under a variety of conditions to provide a working guide for field trials. In typical experiments, glass slides were coated with microencapsulated formulations and exposed under laboratory and field conditions. Bioassay and pheromone release measurements were used for comparative assessment after exposure. We found that capsules located outdoors lost half of their lure content in 10 to 34 days, whereas about 123 days was required under laboratory conditions.

The emission rate measurements showed that, in general, the microcapsule and matrix formulations gave a high release rate for the first few days. Following this period, the rate declined more slowly as a function of aging time. Table II shows some of the data obtained for both emission rates and lure contents for samples aged outdoors in Maryland in spring 1976. Sticker was not added to these test samples.

A much higher percentage of the applied lure was emitted over a 9-week period from the 2% NCR formulation than from the 10% NCR material. The rate of emission did not increase in proportion to the increase in lure content; instead the 10% formulation emitted lure at a relatively high rate for a longer period. After 9 weeks of aging, the 10% NCR formulation emitted lure at 2 to 3 times the rate of the 2% material per milligram of initially applied lure. Therefore the 2% NCR formulation efficiently released its lure during the moth flight season, but the 10% formulation had a longer active lifetime.

The Stauffer formulation listed in Table II was modified to improve its efficiency for field application; a mixture of 3 parts 2% capsules and 1 part 10% capsules (average of 4%) was used for field tests.

The RA-1645 ® sticker (Monsanto Corp., Indian Orchard, Mass.) used with the NCR and MGK materials reduced the emission rate by over 50% when 2% of this sticker was added to the formulations. To minimize this problem, we used only 1% for field applications.

No emission measurements were made on Conrel fibers.

1976 Field Trials for Comparative Evaluation of Formulations

Tests were conducted in June and July by the Animal and Plant Health Inspection Service, the Agricultural Research Service, and the Maryland Department of Agriculture; duplicate experiments were run in Maryland and Massachusetts (21).

The formulations selected for field tests are shown in Table I. The NCR capsules consisted of a plastic-coated, gelatin wall encasing a 3:1 xylene : amyl acetate solution of 2.2% or 11% disparlure; since the wall material is 10% of the

TABLE II

Emission of Lure from Aged Samples

Manufacturer	% Lure in Capsules	Lure Content Measurements: mg lure in test sample at t_o	Lure Content Measurements: mg lure in test sample at 9 wks	% Loss of lure	Emission Rate Measurements: µg/hr ** after aging 4 days	Emission Rate Measurements: µg/hr ** after aging 4 wks	Emission Rate Measurements: µg/hr ** after aging 9 wks
NCR-1975	2	3.7	1.0	73	0.4	0.1	0.005
NCR-1976	2	2.5	0.6	75	0.6	0.2	0.02
NCR-1976	3/4 : 2 1/4 : 10	4.9	1.9	60	0.3	0.2	0.02
NCR-1976	10	9.6	6.8	29	0.2	0.08	0.05
Stauffer *	4	1.5	1.3	13	0.4	0.3	0.2
MGK	2	1.6	0.3	82	0.3	0.1	0.08

* Not the formulation applied in the field; the field formulation contained 3/4 capsules with 2% lure and 1/4 capsules with 10% lure.

** Per mg of lure originally present.

capsule weight, the lure content of the capsules was 2% and 10% respectively. The 4% formulation was a mixture of 3 parts of the 2% formulation with 1 part of the 10% formulation. The capsules were suspended in water containing a thickening agent and an adhesive or sticker to hold the sprayed capsules onto the foliage. The sticker for the 1975 NCR formulation was 1% Rhoplex B-15 ® (Rohm and Haas, Philadelphia, Penn.); that for the 1976 NCR formulations was 1% RA-1645 ® plus 0.1% Triton X-202 ® (Rohm and Haas). The Stauffer formulation was an aqueous suspension of cross-linked polyurea microcapsules of which 75% contained 2.2% disparlure and 25% contained 11% disparlure in xylene; a thickening agent and an adhesive were also present. The MGK was an aqueous slurry of particles of a paraffin wax-inorganic salt matrix containing 2% disparlure; a thickener and an adhesive (same as used in 1976 NCR formulations) were also added. The Conrel fibers were hollow (8 mil ID) plastic fibers, 2.3 cm in length, filled with 30% disparlure in hexane.

Test plots were established in both Maryland (Cecil County) and Massachusetts (near Fall River). The population level in the treated areas was estimated by pre-season counts of egg masses before foliation of trees. In Massachusetts, approximately 2 to 3 egg masses/hectare was found; a much lower population was present in Maryland. Each formulation was applied in each state to 4 replicate plots of 16 ha at a rate of 20 g of lure/ha. Eight check or control plots were established in each state. The incidence of mating in the treated plots was compared with that in the check plots by placing virgin female moths in the field and retrieving them after 3 days to determine the number mated. The recovered insects were dissected in the laboratory to determine whether sperm was present. Any egg masses deposited were collected and examined for the presence of fertile eggs.

The overall results of these tests are given in Table III. The percent reduction in mating is 100 minus the ratio: percent mated in treated plots times 100, divided by percent mated in control plots. The ranking of the seven formulations tested was the same in both test locations although the differences among the top performers were not statistically significant. The best performance was shown by the 1976 2% NCR microcapsule formulation with mating reductions of 98 and 83% respectively, for Maryland and Massachusetts. The 4% NCR formulation was second with 95 and 76% mating reduction for the two states. The 1975-2% NCR microcapsules reduced mating by 80% in Maryland and 68% in Massachusetts; this 80% figure for the 1976 tests is the same as that obtained in trials carried out in Maryland in 1975 over a much larger area (22). This duplication of results was encouraging because it provided an element of continuity in the testing program and confirmed our predictions that modification of this formulation for the 1976 tests would improve its performance. We felt that the improved performance of the 1976 NCR formulations is due at least in part to the new RA-1645

TABLE III

Mating Reduction in 1976 Field Tests

Material	Maryland Tests				Massachusetts Tests			
	No. of moths dissected	No. of moths mated	% Mated	% Reduction in mating	No. of moths dissected	No. of moths mated	% mated	% Reduction in mating
Controls *	260	124	47.7	-	644	315	47.9	-
1976-NCR-2%	101	2	2.0	96	364	29	8.0	83
1976-NCR-4%	121	5	4.1	91	273	31	11.4	76
1976-NCR-10%	149	7	4.7	90	270	37	13.7	71
1975-NCR-2%	91	9	9.9	79	292	45	15.4	68
Conrel	76	7	9.2	81	282	59	20.9	56
Stauffer	128	31	24.2	51	356	105	29.5	38
MGK	132	49	37.1	22	358	129	36.0	25

* 8 Control plots, all formulations 4 plots.

sticker, which proved to be a more effective adhesive than the Rhoplex B-15 used in 1975; the RA-1645 also provided an additional coating to the capsules that reduced the release rate of the lure and thus extended the active life of the capsules. In addition, the smaller average particle size of the 1976 NCR capsules increased the number of capsules per acre and improved adhesion and retention on foliage.

Laboratory tests of all formulations during the field season indicated that the poor performance of the MGK and Stauffer formulations was due at least in part to the rapid loss of lure during the initial 1 to 2 weeks after application, leaving insufficient lure for control during peak mating. Midsummer aging tests indicated that the release rate of the MGK material increased far more as a function of higher outdoor temperatures than did those of the microencapsulated formulations.

It is important to examine the mating figures throughout the season to evaluate the degree of control at the relatively high mid-season populations. Plots of percent mating vs number of days after application for the 1976-NCR-2 and 1976-NCR-4 formulations and for the controls are shown in Figures 2 and 3. A three-point running average was used for the percent mating figures. During the period of peak mating (mid July) even the 2% NCR formulation did not adequately control mating. A second application of the capsules or a initial lure application rate higher than 20 g/ha may be necessary to maintain mating below 10% throughout the field season.

Future field plans will include tests to determine the effect of a second application of the 2% NCR formulation. In addition, application rates significantly higher than the 20 g/ha will be tested.

Discussion

Although air permeation with pheromone presents a potential method of controlling some pest populations, there are many difficulties to be overcome before the technique becomes economical and practical. Our aim was to provide a sprayable formulation that would successfully disrupt mating throughout the flight period of the gypsy moth in the forest environment. This objective met with limited success, and we shall continue our research to improve the performance of our controlled release formulations. Optimization of pheromone formulations will depend on a number of factors. The first of these is the behavior of the insect during the flight period, and the second is the physico-chemical behavior of a controlled-release formulation in a forest environment.

McDonough (14) has discussed the theoretical case in which a formulation releases pheromone at a rate proportional to the amount remaining (a first order process) and has given an equation

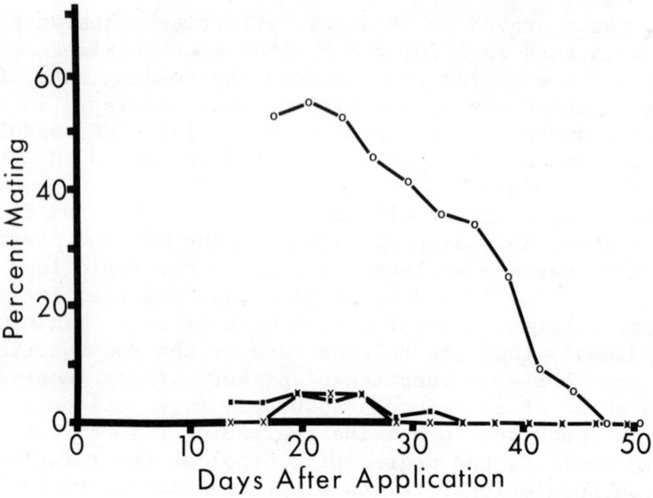

Figure 2. Maryland tests: ○—○ *control;* ×—× *1976–NCR-2;* ■—■ *1976–NCR-4*

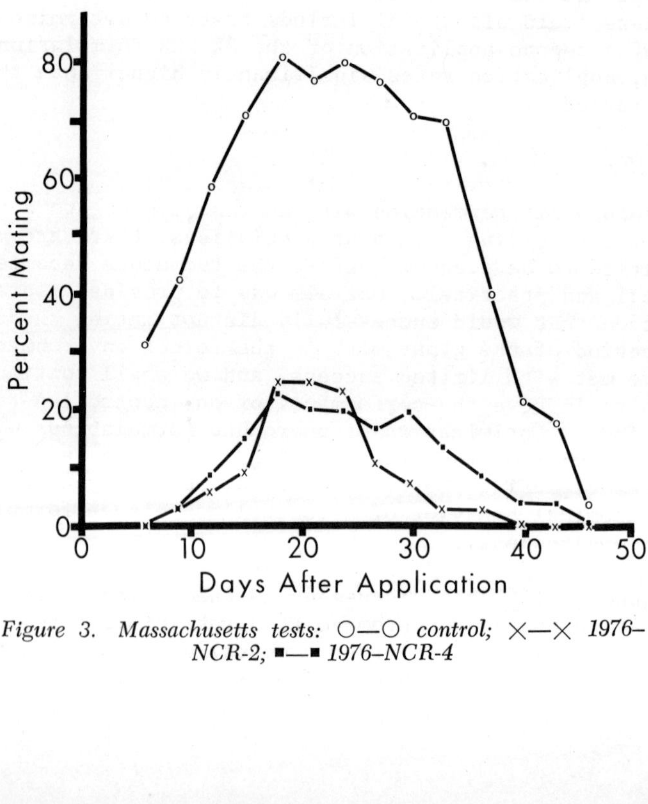

Figure 3. Massachusetts tests: ○—○ *control;* ×—× *1976–NCR-2;* ■—■ *1976–NCR-4*

for the application level of the pheromone (C_o) based on a desired half-life period, $t_{1/2}$

$$C_o = Re^{kt}/k$$

$$\text{where } k = (\ln 2)\ t_{1/2}$$

(R is the minimum release rate, t is the period of control desired for the application, and e is the natural base of logarithms).

From data on the codling moth, (Laspeyresia pomonella (L.)) solution of this equation gives a figure for C_o of 13.1 g/ha for a 30-day period of control. However, this theoretical treatment neglects the wide variation in environmental conditions to which the formulation is exposed. Our own experiments showed that temperature and wind velocity had a considerable effect on the emission rate. Rain and sunlight also contributed towards unpredictable changes in the lifetime of the formulation, and we found that the time in which the lure content had decreased by 50% varied greatly depending on the conditions of exposure.

Microencapsulated formulations of a volatile solute in a solvent should show predictable release characteristics for a period after an initial burst of pheromone emission, because in theory the rate of emission is controlled by diffusion of solute through the capsule wall. However, in practice, rapid loss of volatile solvent results in behavior unlike that theoretically predicted. Our findings were paralleled in laboratory studies of emission rate by Roelofs et al. (23) who found that the rate of pheromone emission dropped from 0.7% per day to 0.02% by the 16th day when only 3.7% of a mixture of 11-tetradecenyl acetates had been released by a microencapsulated formulation.

In the forest, the situation is even more complex. Air measurements of disparlure concentrations showed that a layering effect occurred. Most of the pheromone appeared to be near the ground and there was a considerable difference between concentrations measured at 0.5 m and 15.0 m height. Measurement of disparlure in air from a formulation applied to a flat, grass plot showed that over a period of 30 days, only 2% of the applied disparlure could be accounted for in the air (24). Thus in addition to the air, there are probably other "sinks" which rapidly take up disparlure released by the formulation. We suggest that the surfaces of the soil, leaves, and plants probably adsorb the pheromone rapidly. The close resemblance of disparlure to the long chain hydrocarbon structures common in plant leaf waxes would be expected to favor its ready adsorption and retention by such surfaces.

Experience in fumigation has taught that air permeation is best achieved when volatile chemicals are not highly sorbed by the substrate and that special techniques may be required to improve the distribution of heavier-than-air vapors. These factors will be important in the efficient use of pheromones, and it seems likely that the ability of a forest or plant surface to adsorb pheromone will significantly affect performance of a controlled-release formulation applied uniformly to foliage.

Literature Cited

1. Beroza, M., "Pest Management with Insect Sex Attractants and Other Behavior-controlling Chemicals",M. Beroza, ed. ACS Symposium Series No. 23. American Chemical Society, Washington, D.C. 1976 pp 99-118.
2. Roelofs, W. L., Miller, J. R., Baker, T. C., in "Perspectives in Forest Entomology", J. F. Anderson and H. K. Kaya, eds. Academic Press, New York, 1976. pp 111-125
3. Knipling, E. F., Environ. Health Perspectives 14, 145-152 (1976).
4. Beroza, M., Knipling, E. F., Science 177, 19-27 (1972).
5. Pest Control: An Assessment of Present and Alternative Technologies." Vol. IV "Forest Pest Control. National Academy of Sciences, Washington, D. C. 1975, pp 114-120.
6. Leonard, D. E., Ann. Rev. Entomol. 19, 197-229 (1974).
7. Cardé, R. T., Doane, C. C., Roelofs, W. L. Can. Entomol. 106, 479-484 (1974).
8. Iwaki, S., Marumo, S., Saito, T., Yamada, M., Katagiri, K., J. Amer. Chem.Soc. 96, 7842-7843 (1974).
9. Yamada, M., Saito, T., Katagiri, K., Iwaki, S., Marumo, S., J. Insect Physiol. 22, 755-761 (1976).
10. Vité, J. P., Klimetzek, D., Loskant, G., Hedden, R., Mori, K., Naturwissenschaften 63, 582-583 (1976).
11. Plimmer, J. R., Schwalbe, C. P., Paszek, E. C., Bierl, B. A., Webb, R. E., Marumo, S., Iwaki, S. (in preparation).
12. Mori, K., Takigawa, T., Matsui, M., Tetrahedron Lett. 3953-3956 (1976).
13. Beroza, M., Agr. Chem. 15, 37-40 (1960).
14. McDonough, L. M. presented at 172nd ACS National Meeting, Aug. 30-Sept. 3, 1976; Environ. Entomol. (submitted).
15. Plimmer, J. R., Bierl, B. A. DeVilbiss, E. D., Smith, B. L. Proc. Internatl. Controlled Release Pestic. Symp., Akron, Ohio, 1976. In press.
16. Mastro, V. C., Richerson, J. V., Cameron, E. A., Environ. Entomol. 6, 128-132 (1977).
17. Beroza, M., Paszek, E. C., DeVilbiss, E. D., Bierl, B. A., Tardif, J. G. R., Environ. Entomol. 4, 712-714 (1975).
18. Bierl, B. A., DeVilbiss, E. D., Plimmer, J. R., in "Controlled Release Polymeric Formulations", D. R. Paul and F. W. Harris, eds. ACS Symposium Series No. 33. American Chemical Society, Washington, D. C. 1976. pp. 265-272.
19. Beroza, M., Stevens, L. J., Bierl, B. A., Philips, F. M., Tardif, J. G. R. Environ. Entomol. 2, 1051-1057 (1973).

20. Bierl, B. A., DeVilbiss, E. D., Proc. Internatl. Controlled Release Pesti. Symp., Dayton, Ohio, 1975. pp. 230-246.
21. Schwalbe, C. P., Webb, R. E., McComb, C., Dull, C., Altman, R, Bierl, B. A. and Plimmer, J. R., (in preparation).
22. Webb, R. E., Plimmer, J. R., Bierl, B. A., Schwalbe, C. P., (unpublished results).
23. Roelofs, W. L., Carde, R. T., Taschenberg, E. F., Weires, R. W., Jr., ACS Symposium Series No. 23 (1976), 75-87.
24. Caro, J. H., Bierl, B. A., Freeman, H. P., Glotfelty, D. E., Turner, B. C., presented at the 173rd ACS National Meeting, New Orleans, Louisiana, March 21-25, 1977.

Acknowledgement:

The work reported herein was funded in part by the U.S.D.A. Expanded Gypsy Moth Research & Development program.

16

Controlled Release Formulations of Insect Growth Regulators and Pheromones—Evaluation Methods and Field Test Results

J. W. YOUNG, T. M. GRAVES, and R. CURTIS

Zoecon Corp., 975 California Ave., Palo Alto, Calif. 94304

M. M. FURNISS

Forest Service, U.S. Department of Agriculture, Moscow, Idaho 83843

This third section of our Symposium has been entitled "Utility of Controlled Release Pesticides." It is my intention to share with you three instances in my experience in which controlled release techniques provided the key element of utility. In each case, the availability of a controlled delivery system made a product possible which would otherwise have been impossible. I will attempt to outline for you the formulation screening procedures which were used, and to indicate with some field data the effectiveness of the final delivery system.

Mosquito Larvicide

To properly introduce this first topic, I will need to describe briefly the mode of action of the active ingredient since that has an important bearing on the nature of the problem.

The factors controlling insect growth and metamorphosis have been the subject of biological investigations since early in this century. By the 1960s, it was known that particular glands secreted substances which initiated the molting process in insects, and which controlled the complex series of metamorphoses from egg, through larva and pupa, to adult (1). One hormone, secreted by a small pair of glands called the corpora allata, was known to be responsible for the maintenance of preadult characters throughout the immature life stages of insects. It is the lowering of titre of this material, called Juvenile Hormone, which allows for metamorphosis of immature insects into adults. It had been speculated that treatment of an insect with Juvenile Hormone at a time when the hormone should have been absent should cause it to carry larval characteristics into the next developmental stage -- a derangement of the normal process which would in all likelihood be lethal. In 1967, a research group at the University of Wisconsin announced the structure of a Juvenile Hormone (JH I) (2). A closely related structure was identified soon afterward (JH II) (3). The third natural Juvenile Hormone (JH III) was discovered in our own laboratories using a novel tissue culture technique (4).

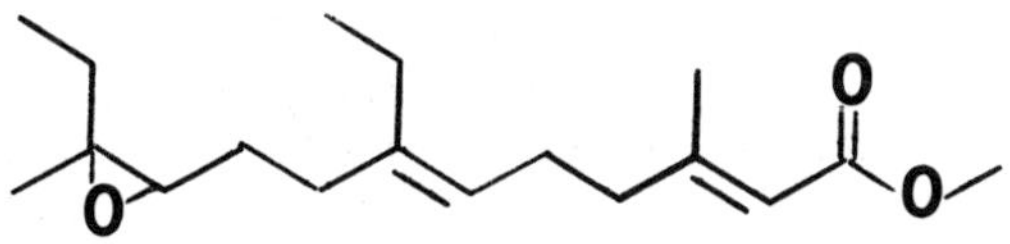

JH I

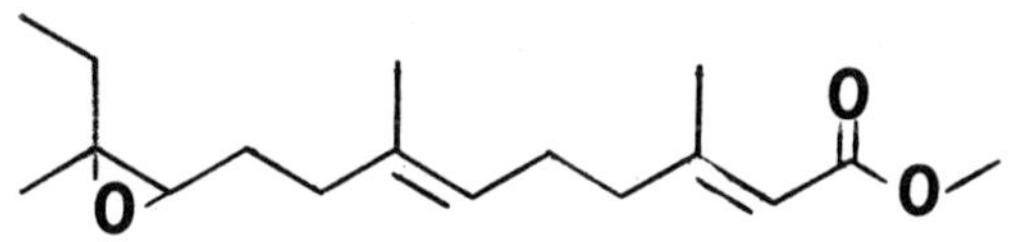

JH II

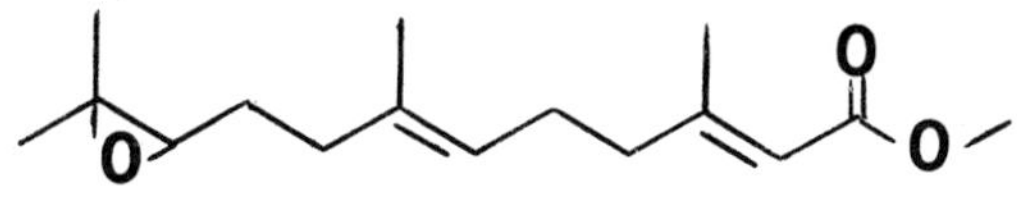

JH III

In 1968, Zoecon was formed with one specific immediate goal, among others, of developing from these discoveries a new, hopefully selective, insect control agent.

One of the first of the Juvenile Hormone-type materials prepared in Zoecon's laboratories which appeared feasible for commercialization now carries the common name "methoprene" and our trademark "ALTOSID®."

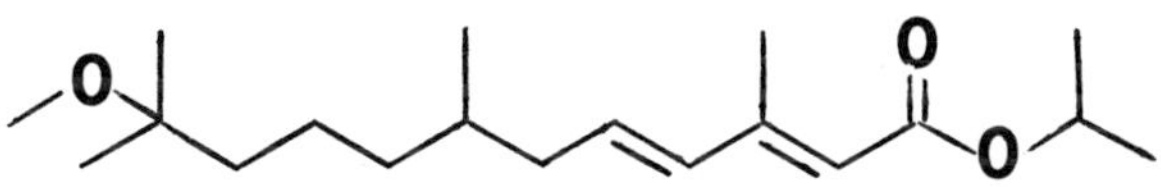

methoprene
ALTOSID® IGR

Because of their mode of action, methoprene and chemicals like it are now called "Insect Growth Regulators" (IGR). The effects of treatment with IGRs vary somewhat from one insect to another, but in general, insect sensitivity to the compounds occurs late in larval development, with mortality due to morphological effects and physiological imperfections delayed until the last larval instar or the pupal stage.

One of the first applications of methoprene which we explored, once its biological characteristics were known, was its use as a mosquito larvicide. The mode of action of IGRs on mosquito larvae is very different from classical insecticides. Rather than toxicity to larvae soon after treatment, IGR-treated larvae develop normally through the pupal stage, but then fail to emerge as adults. This unusual sort of activity has made necessary several new developments in field trial evaluation methods. It was not possible to simply count dead vs. live larvae in order to gauge the effect of the treatment. In some cases, treated water containing larvae was sampled in the field, brought into the laboratory, and the larvae observed for inhibition of adult emergence. In other trials, larvae were introduced into treated water either in the laboratory or in specially designed floating cages.

Soon after we began field testing of methoprene, we noted rapid degradation -- the inverse of the problem encountered with sometimes too-persistent conventional pesticides. The active ingredient was simply not lasting long enough under field exposure conditions to be biologically effective. Chemical analysis quickly confirmed that at least two different reactions were occuring which converted methoprene to inactive materials (5). The first of these processes was found to be rapid ultraviolet light-induced isomerization to the much less active 2Z,4E isomer (B below).

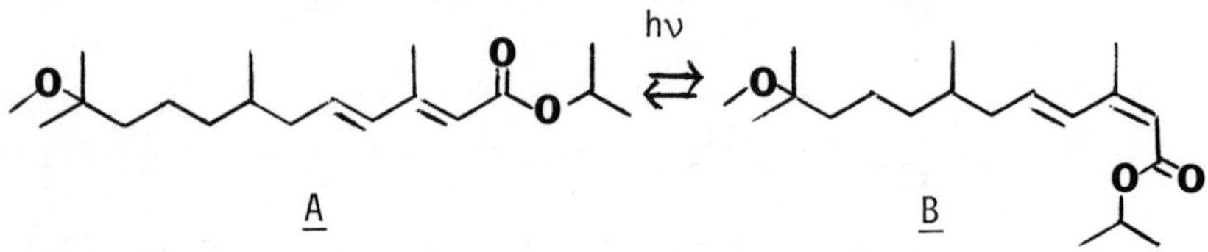

Table I shows that a second process, involving decomposition to nonisomeric products, occurs simultaneously.

Table I

Percent Methoprene Isomers Remaining After Exposure to Sunlight

	% B	% A	% A+B
Initial	10	90	100
1 hour	30	65	95
2 hours	39	50	89
4 hours	36	42	78
8 hours	27	35	62

It has since been determined (5) that sunlight initiates rapid decay to the biologically inactive decomposition products shown below.

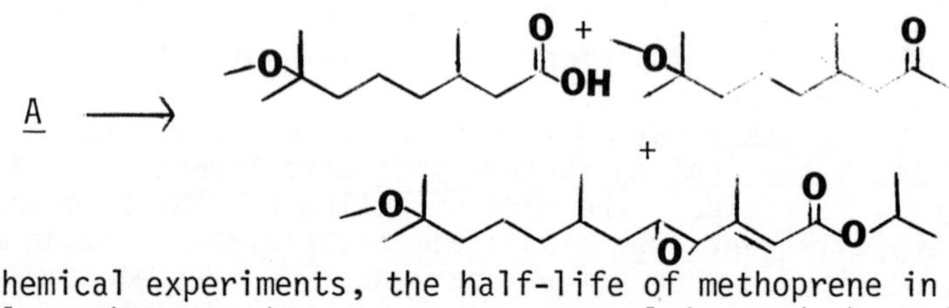

In these chemical experiments, the half-life of methoprene in sunlight was less than one day as an aqueous emulsion and about four hours as a thin film on glass.

The rapid decomposition indicated in Table I merely served as chemical confirmation of the complete failure of conventional formulations of methoprene in early field tests, although the same formulations had been highly effective in laboratory tests. Even though we were dealing with floodwater mosquitoes and synchronous populations, the susceptibility of fourth instar larvae to methoprene required pinpoint application timing for effectiveness.

A formulation was thus needed which protected the active ingredient and released it in biologically active form, but did not leave residues beyond those required for effectiveness (see Table II).

Table II

Project Goals -- ALTOSID Mosquito Formulation

1. Decrease rate of isomerization to the less active isomer.
2. Decrease rate of oxidative degradation.
3. Achieve efficient use of active ingredient -- must be biologically effective for 4-10 days.
4. Predictable residues.

In preparing candidate formulations, the principal variables which we explored are those shown in Table III. Formulations were first screened in laboratory glassware. Aqueous dilutions were subjected to aging under artificial light, and then infested with sensitive fourth instar larvae (6). Later tests were conducted similarly, but in series of outdoor ponds either one meter^2 or 130 meters^2 in size (7). Biological testing revealed most significant gains in effective lifetime of the active ingredient with a polyamide formulation which we now call ALTOSID SR-10. The product is an aqueous dispersion of microparticles in the 1-10 micron range, and contains 10% active ingredient. Our formulation procedure does not yield true microcapsules -- oil droplets surrounded by a film of polymeric wall material. ALTOSID SR-10 appears on microscopic examination to be a matrix which is sponge-like in cross-section.

Table III

Formulation Variables

1. Capsule wall/matrix material
2. Ratio of polymer to active ingredient
3. Degree of cross-linking
4. Particle size
5. Particle specific gravity

The effect of this formulation on the rate of isomerization to the 2Z,4E isomer (B, Table I), is shown in Figure 1. Although that process is not stopped altogether, its rate is substantially decreased relative to that of unprotected material supplied as an emulsifiable concentrate (E.C.) formulation. Methoprene has a water solubility of 1.4 parts per million (ppm). Its threshold of biological activity and the level of detection by our residue methods are both about 1 part per billion (ppb). Figure 2 shows the cumulative effect on the product's lifetime of the decrease both in isomerization rate and in rate of oxidative degradation.

Many of our early formulation screening experiments involved twofold evaluation procedures. Water was sampled and analyzed chemically for residues of methoprene after various aging periods. At the same time, biological performance was monitored by placing sensitive fourth instar mosquito larvae in the treated water. We repeatedly saw instances of complete biological effectiveness of the treatment while no methoprene was chemically detectable. It was not until we began to note the time of day at which samples were taken for chemical analysis that a pattern emerged. That pattern is shown in Figure 3. Our rationalization of this result is that the rate of decomposition of released methoprene exceeds the release rate itself during the sunlit hours of the day. During the cool, dark hours, release of the active ingredient continues and establishes a biologically efficacious pool of methoprene.

Analytical Methods. Evaluation of the efficiency of various microencapsulation procedures is a problem which has persisted throughout this and all similar projects with which we have been involved. It occurs in the initial stages of product development when one needs a rapid means of evaluating the effect of formulation variables, and persists throughout the lifetime of the product as a vital aspect of quality control. The problem, simply stated, is not too different from one encountered by high energy physicists -- in measuring this particular property of the particle, one cannot avoid changing the nature of the particle itself. We have arrived at a method which, although it undoubtedly does suffer from this defect, serves the purpose of yielding highly reproducible data in a relatively rapid fashion. The method itself is summarized in Table IV, while the results of two representative analyses are shown in Figure 4. At short time intervals, the curve obtained is very nonlinear, which is undoubtedly due to dissolution of unencapsulated material along with a quantity at or near the surface of the particles. At longer intervals, however, we find that with the proper choice of extracting solvent, very reproducible straight lines are obtained which allow the characterization of the particular batch of product.

For simplicity, the term "encapsulation efficiency" is employed here. The method as outlined appears to have validity in a wide range of formulations -- true encapsulates as well as matrix systems such as ALTOSID SR-10.

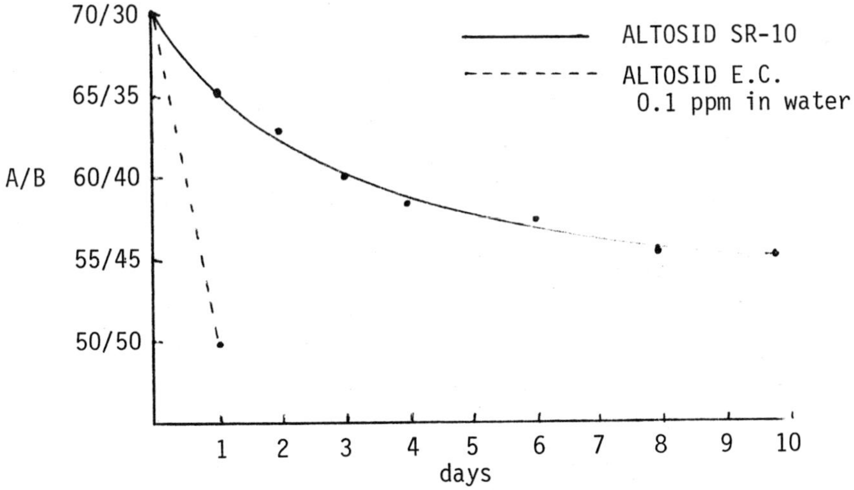

Figure 1. Change of methoprene isomer ratio—sunlight

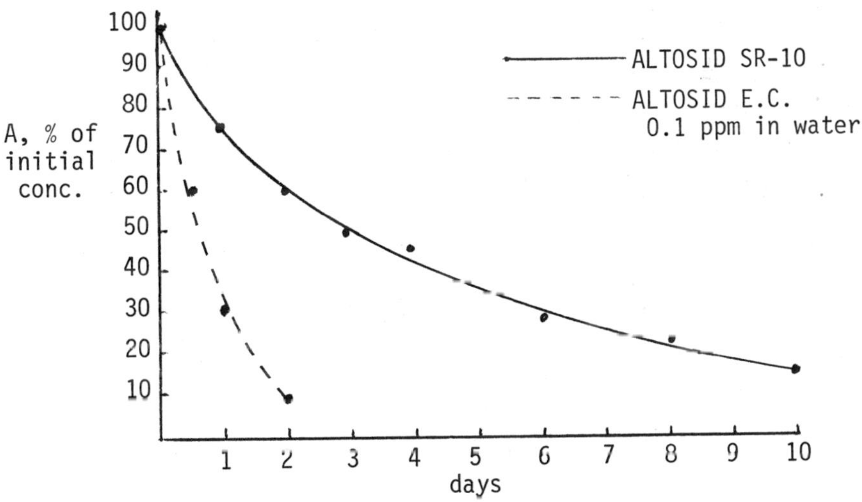

Figure 2. Methoprene decomposition—sunlight

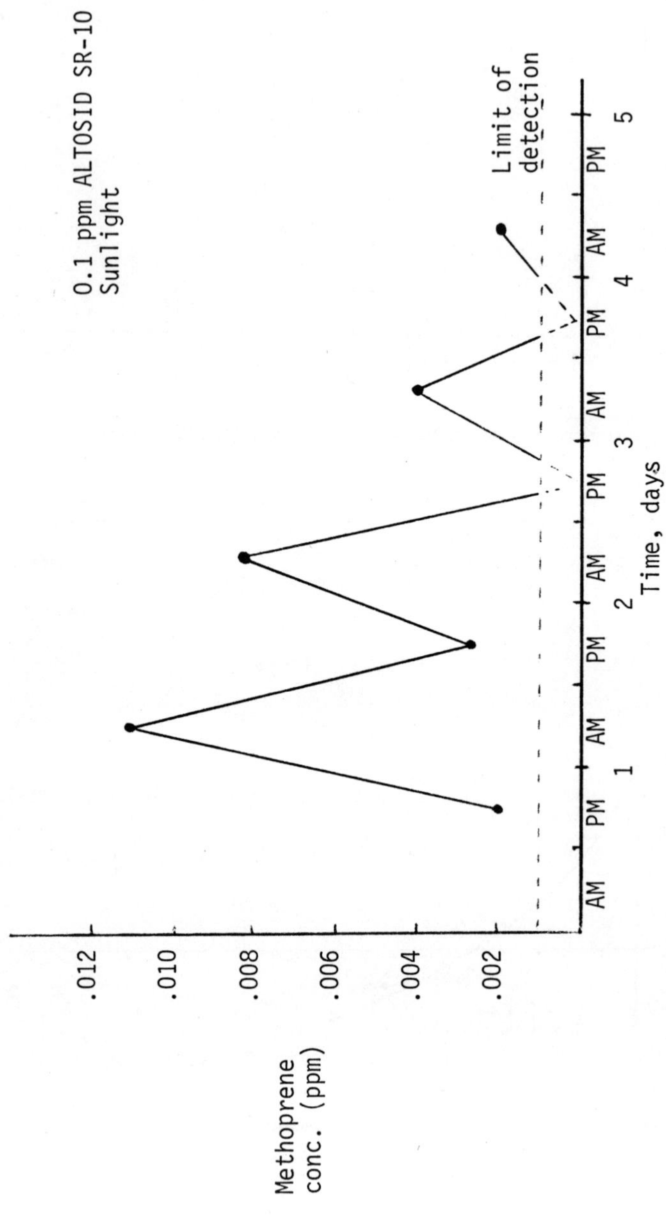

Figure 3. Effect of sampling time on methoprene residues detected

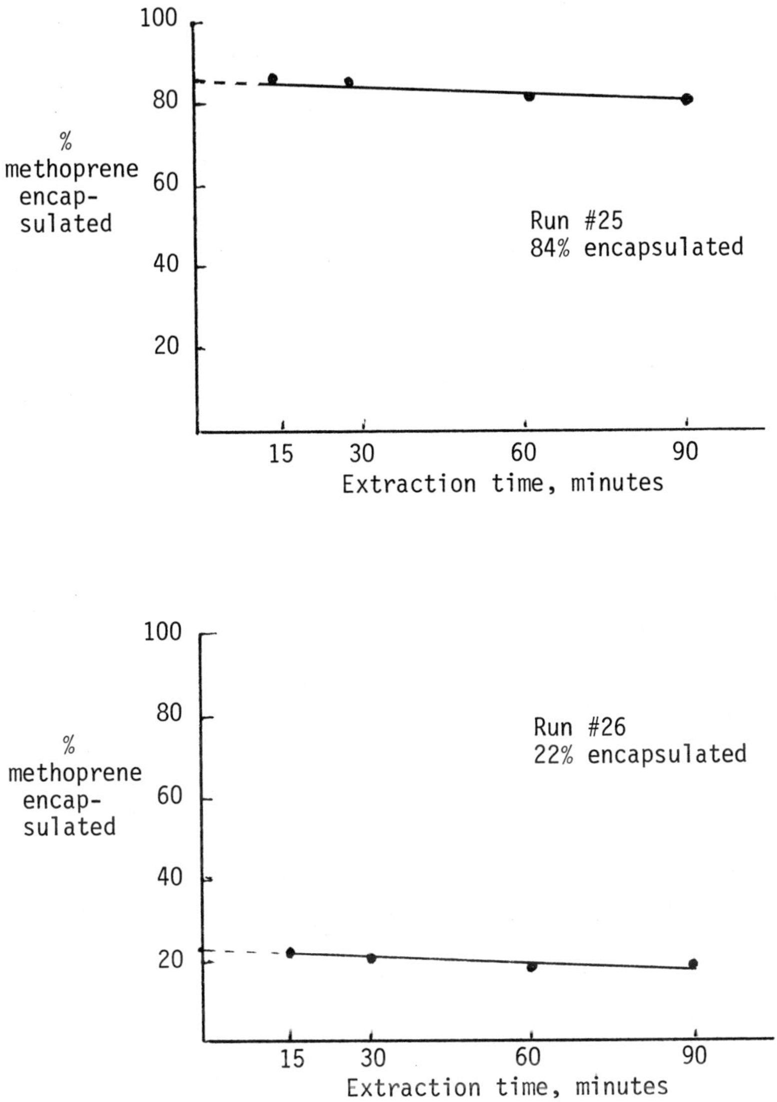

Figure 4. Encapsulation efficiency

Table IV

Analytical Method -- Encapsulation Efficiency

Step 1: Analyze total A.I. available. High shear mixing to rupture particles -- strong solvent system.

Step 2: Mild extraction procedure

- A) Dilute controlled release formulation in water.
- B) Add solvent containing internal standard for GLC analysis. Solvent chosen is solvent for active ingredient, nonsolvent for polymer, immiscible in water.
- C) Shake the sample containing the solvent on a wrist-shaker. Remove aliquots of the supernatant solvent for analysis at standard intervals.
- D) Analyze (by GLC or other suitable means) for % active ingredient in the solvent.

Step 3: Determine % encapsulated A.I.

- A) Plot X vs. extraction time.

$$X = 100 - \left[\frac{\text{wt. detected}}{\text{total wt. available}} \times 100\right]$$

- B) Extrapolate to zero time.

Fly Control -- Poultry Feed Through

Another area investigated very actively with methoprene is that of fly control in poultry houses. In caged laying hen operations in particular, flies present serious nuisance and disease vector problems. Managers of these operations are forced to follow very rigid programs of manure clean-out and frequent insecticide sprays to control their fly populations. Because of the extraordinary safety of ALTOSID, we felt it could be incorporated into the feed rations of the birds. If it emerged intact in the manure, and any fly larvae developing there would not emerge as adults.

In preliminary tests, small groups of laying hens were fed with a ration treated with technical methoprene over a wide range of concentrations. The manure was infested with housefly larvae, and the various treatments were scored for percent inhibition of adult emergence. The results are shown in Table V. In this and in subsequent work, the level of methoprene in the manure required for effective control fell in the range of 1-2 ppm.

Table V

Rate of Methoprene in Poultry Feed, ppm	Percent Inhibition of Adult House Fly Emergence	Level of Methoprene Detected in Manure, ppm
10	68	
25	81	1.0
50	96	1.5
75	98	
100	99+	2.5
125	100	
200	100	
400	100	

Economic analysis indicated to us that the market would bear the cost of the product only if the level of methoprene to be incorporated into the feed could be reduced to 10 ppm or less and that >95% fly control was required. These factors, then, defined the target for formulation work. When fed as technical material, the amount of methoprene excreted intact was on the order of 3%. It was our task to formulate the product to yield a five- to tenfold increase in feed-through efficiency.

Formulation screening involved both chemical and biological evaluation of each candidate. Not only was it necessary to determine the level of active ingredient present in the poultry manure, but its bioavailability had to be ascertained. Small groups of hens were fed rations containing 10 ppm methoprene in a variety of formulations, and manure was sampled 10 and 14 days after treatment. Part of the sample was inocculated with house fly larvae, and methoprene residues determined by chemical analysis were compared with the percent inhibition of adult fly emergence. Figure 5 shows the results for several formulations tested early in the program (numbers 1 through 7) and for the formulation ALTOSID PS-10 which ultimately emerged as suitable for further testing (number 8). It should be noted that the biological data indicates considerably greater efficacy than would be expected at these residue levels. This probably reflects the somewhat idealized conditions of the laboratory experiment. The excellent performance of ALTOSID PS-10 in small-scale efficacy experiments prompted us to file for an experimental permit registration to allow expanded testing. Under the experimental permit, testing involved extremely large numbers of birds in several states.

The results of two of the many trials conducted under the experimental permit are shown at the bottom of Table VI. While in 1974, the treatment yielded 90% or greater control in most instances, effectiveness in full-house trials a year later was variable and much lower.

Sample #	Formulation Type	10 Days Residue (ppm)	10 Days % Control Avg. of 3 Reps	14 Days Residue (ppm)	14 Days % Control Avg. of 3 Reps
1	Untreated Control	-	25	-	12
2	Technical	0.36	93	0.39	92
3	Fumed Silica	0.22	84	0.29	71
4	Calcium Silicate	0.21	97	0.26	71
5	Calcium Silicate/ Polyamide Coating	0.62	98	0.94	97
6	Celite	0.55	96	0.62	98
7	Celite/Polyurea Coating	0.39	98	0.32	92
8	ALTOSID PS-10	2.00	100	2.50	100

Figure 5. Formulation screening: poultry feed-through—10 ppm in feed

Table VI

ALTOSID PS-10 Manure Residue & Efficacy

Date	Test Location	Feeding Rate	Formulation	Percent Control	ppm in Manure
1974	California	10 ppm	PS-10	97	1.2
1974	California	10 ppm	PS-10	95	1.6
1974	California	10 ppm	PS-10	98	2.0
1974	Texas	10 ppm	PS-10	90	1.4
1974	Texas	10 ppm	PS-10	89	1.6
1975	California	10 ppm	PS-10	42	1.7
1975	Texas	10 ppm	PS-10	39	1.5

The contrasting results are undoubtedly related to the difference in evaluation techniques employed. In small trials, it was necessary to judge the effectiveness of the treatment by monitoring inhibition of adult fly emergence from small closed containers of manure. In larger tests, movement of the natural population of fly larvae was not restricted, and evaluation was made by actual fly counts on a whole ranch or whole house basis.

The failure of large tests to demonstrate the commercial viability of this product results from failure of the IGR to act during early stages of larval development. It was observed that fly larvae developing in wet areas in the manure tend to move shortly before pupation to dried areas -- away from freshly deposited droppings. Since this time in the life cycle of the fly coincides with the period of sensitivity to the IGR, the time of exposure to the active ingredient is insufficient. In many cases, this phenomenon was aggravated in 1975 by an unusually rainy fly season.

Although these results were disappointing, they serve to illustrate an important point. No matter how well one believes to have designed small-scale experiments, the jump to commercial-sized testing invariably brings into play a number of variables not present in the smaller trials.

Anti-Aggregative Pheromone -- Douglas Fir Bark Beetle

The Douglas Fir Bark Beetle infests Douglas fir forests throughout much of the Northwestern United States. Its population occasionally reaches epidemic proportions, especially in trees weakened by windthrow or disease. It was discovered in 1971 (8) that the frass of the female beetle contains a pheromone, 3-methyl-2-cyclohexen-1-one (MCH), which was later shown (9,10) to have anti-aggregative effects on adult beetles. In 1974, Furniss et al (11) reported on field trials with felled host trees which showed that, when released optimally, the pheromone served to reduce beetle attacks upon susceptible trees by 96%. The pheromone was dispensed in this experiment as neat material from small metal canisters mounted at even spacings around the tree on wooden stakes. This trial served to demonstrate the effectiveness of the treatment, and refined the optimum rate of pheromone release to a narrow range.

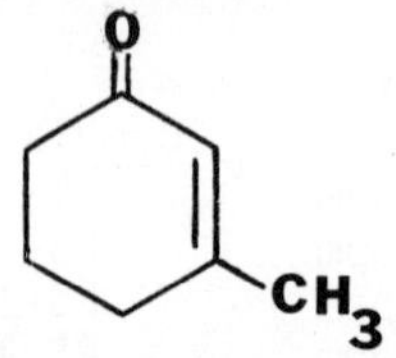

3-methyl-2-cyclohexen-1-one

We became involved at this stage, and began work aimed at developing a formulation for season-long release of MCH, a highly volatile and water soluble material. The properties of the formulation would ideally match those outlined in Table VII.

Table VII

Goals -- MCH Formulation Project

1. Release MCH at rate of 0.1-1.3 grams/acre/day
2. Effective for 30-60 days
3. Suitable for application by air -- must penetrate forest canopy
4. Biodegradable
5. Nontoxic
6. Low cost

The first step in our program was the development of a release rate method suitable for laboratory screening of the many formulations which would be necessary (12). The method as it developed involved the use of tritium-labeled MCH. The formulation to be tested was placed in a modified flask (13) fitted with inlet and outlet for carrier gas flow. To the outlet of the flask was attached a small glass tube packed with 0.25 grams of Porapak® QS (50-80 mesh) (14). Dry nitrogen carrier gas was passed through the flask and trapping column for one hour at a rate of 175 ml/minute. The trapping column was then removed, and the ^{3}H-MCH released from the formulation was eluted into a scintillation vial with 10 cc's of hexane. Scintillation fluid was added to the vial, and the ^{3}H-MCH content was determined directly by scintillation counting.

Formulations were aged at ambient temperature and relative humidity for up to 60 days on paper-lined steel trays stacked in a forced draft fume hood with a constant air flow through the stack of trays of 150 cu. ft./min. Formulations were sampled for release rate determination at the beginning of the aging period and weekly thereafter until the rate of release of ^{3}H-MCH fell below 0.5 micrograms/hour.

Treatment	Method[1]	Douglas Fir Beetle Attacks	Brood
Coated Molecular Sieve Granules	P	[3]0.1**	1**
Liquid Standard	P	0.2**	4**
Polyamide Granules A	B	0.3*	33 NS
Polyamide Granules B	B	0.4*	7**
Polyamide Granules C	B	0.6*	26 NS
Coated Molecular Sieve Granules	B	1.7 NS	51 NS
Coated Molecular Sieve Granules[2]	B	3.5 NS	42 NS
Control	-	4.8	45
Coated Kobrite Granules	B	4.9 NS	54 NS

[1]P = in cans on stakes 4 ft. above ground, 10 by 10 ft. spacing; B = broadcast by hand.

[2]Applied at a rate of 1/10 that of the other granules.

[3]Difference from control is significant at the 0.01 (**), 0.5 level (*), or not significant (NS).

Figure 6. Density (no/ft²) of Douglas Fir beetle attacks and brood by treatment

This formulation screening method was convenient and rapid enough to allow testing of relatively large numbers of formulation systems. We conducted release rate tests with about 70 different formulations (several of them replicated three times). Release rates were run at an average of five aging intervals for each formulation. Most systems were eliminated from further consideration after the first few weeks of screening, when the rate of release of MCH fell below 0.5 micrograms/hour. Twelve formulations, however, showed promise and maintained a rate of release of ^{3}H-MCH close to or above 1 microgram/hour for 30-60 days. These formulations were evaluated by an independent laboratory (13), and eventually five formulations were selected for field testing.

The details of this field test will be reported separately (12). In general, the procedure involved treatment of isolated, felled, host trees with the formulations at a rate of 38 grams MCH per acre. The stake-mounted cans containing unformulated MCH served as a standard. Each treatment was replicated three times, and six untreated control plots were reserved. Treatment was made prior to the first beetle flight in April, and final evaluation of treatments was made in mid-August. The results of the test are shown in Figure 6.

As indicated in Figure 6, one of the formulations applied to the ground by broadcast method gave excellent results -- indistinguishable from the standard treatment. This material, a dimer acid polyamide granular formulation (3-8 mesh), was judged sufficiently effective to be used in large-scale trials in areas of natural windthrow. These trials are still in the planning stage.

One other formulation, 13X molecular sieve granules coated with a wax/polymer system, gave excellent performance when protected in metal cans on stakes above the ground, but failed entirely when broadcast on the ground. It is likely that exposure to the high rainfall of the area and constant contact with the moist forest floor extracted the pheromone from that formulation.

Acknowledgements

The authors thank Robert Lowe and Loren Dunham for advice and assistance in the Analytical Chemistry aspects of this work. Edward Wenik developed the assay method for encapsulation efficiency, and Kenneth Horwege provided valuable technical assistance on all of the projects discussed.

The MCH formulation work was funded by the U.S.D.A., Forest Service Contract Number 12-11-205-09.

Literature Cited

1. Wigglesworth, V.B., "The Principles of Insect Physiology," Sixth Edition, E.P. Dutton & Co., New York, 1965.

2. Röller, H., Dahm, K.N., Sweeley, C.C., and Trost, B.M., Angew. Chem. Internat. Ed., (1967), 6, 179.

3. Meyer, A.S., Schneiderman, H.A., Hanzmann, E., Proc. Nat. Acad. Sci. USA, (1968), 60, 853.

4. Judy, K.J., Schooley, D.A., Dunham, L.L., Hall, M.S., Bergot, B.J., and Siddall, J.B., Proc. Nat. Acad. Sci. USA, (1973), 70, 1509.

5. Quistad, G.B., Staiger, L.E., and Schooley, D.A., J. Agr. Food Chem., (1975), 23, 299.

6. Schaefer, C.H., and Wilder, W.H., J. Econ. Ent., (1972), 65, 1066.

7. Schaefer, C.H., and Wilder, W.H., J. Econ. Ent., (1973), 66, 913.

8. Kinzer, G.W., Fentiman, A.F. Jr., Foltz, R.L., Rudinsky, J.A., J. Econ. Ent., (1971), 64, 970.

9. Rudinsky, J.A., Furniss, M.M., Kline, L.N., and Schmitz, R.F., Can. Entomol., (1972), 104, 815.

10. Furniss, M.M., Kline L.N., Schmitz, R.F., and Rudinsky, J.A., Ann. Entomol. Soc. Amer., (1972), 65, 1227.

11. Furniss, M.M., Daterman, G.E., Kline, L.N., McGregor, M.D., Trostle, G.C., Pettinger, L.F., and Kudinsky, J.A., Can. Entomol., (1974), 106, 381.

12. Furniss, M.M., Young, J.W., McGregor, M.D., Livingston, R.L, and Hamel, D.R., Can. Entomol., (1977), in press.

13. Look, M., Chem. Ecol., (1976), 2, 481.

14. The use of Porapak QS was suggested (private communication) by Dr. James Trudell, Stanford University.
See also Byrne, K.J., Gore, W.E., Pearce, G.T., and Silverstein, R.M., J. Chem. Ecol., (1975), 1, 1.

INDEX